12 SECRETS OF DIVINE Health

12 SECRETS OF DIVINE Health

Nicole Y. Edwards, DO
Family Medicine Physician
Founder and Owner of
Abundant Life Concierge

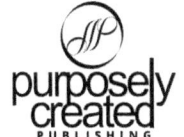

12 SECRETS OF DIVINE HEALTH

Published by Purposely Created Publishing Group™
Copyright © 2018 Nicole Edwards

All rights reserved.

No part of this book may be reproduced, distributed or transmitted in any form by any means, graphic, electronic, or mechanical, including photocopy, recording, taping, or by any information storage or retrieval system, without permission in writing from the publisher, except in the case of reprints in the context of reviews, quotes, or references.

Limit of Liability / Disclaimer of Warranty: While the publisher and author have used their best efforts in preparing this book, they make no representations or warranties with the respect to the accuracy or completeness of the contents of this book and specifically disclaim any implied warranties of fitness for a particular purpose. No warranty may be created or extended by sales representatives or written sales materials. The advice and strategies contained herein may not be suitable for your situation. You should consult with a doctor where appropriate. Neither the publisher nor author shall be liable for any loss or damages including but not limited to special, incidental, consequential or other damages.

Printed in the United States of America
ISBN: 978-1-948400-63-3

Special discounts are available on bulk quantity purchases by book clubs, associations and special interest groups. For details email: sales@publishyourgift.com or call (888) 949-6228.

For information logon to:
www.PublishYourGift.com

Dedication

This book is dedicated to my loving husband, Superior, and children, Ellington and Tatum, who have sacrificed so much for me and continue to love me despite my head in a computer or a book times when I could've been with them. I love you all to life; you are my why. You are why I live, breathe, and have my being, and I will continue to love and live for you all daily. I pray that my children learn from my example how to have a great work ethic, but never forget their family and why they work hard.

I also dedicate this book to my father Pastor Joseph C. Phillips, Jr. Your life has been a blueprint for me: not only for positive things, but even the things you taught me as I watched you work yourself almost to death. You taught me how to work hard, but I've also learned how to better my life and take care of myself first. Abundant Life Concierge was given life when you almost lost yours, and now I strive to take care of Pastors so that no other Pastor's Kid (PK) has to watch their parent give until it hurts. All Pastors give some, but some give all. I'm glad that you're still here to teach others how to give and how to maintain their health and wellness.

I also dedicate this book to my mother Cora E. Phillips, who taught me everything I know about how to be a working wife and mother. If I can be half of the woman and mother you are, then those around me will be so blessed.

This book is in loving memory of Neil and Iona Martin, who modeled a healthy God-fearing lifestyle for me every day. I love you and thank you for the legacy you have passed to me. I pray I make you proud every day.

Table of Contents

Introduction 1

CHAPTER 1:
Meditate Daily 7

CHAPTER 2:
Eat More Fruits and Vegetables 17

CHAPTER 3:
Exercise More 33

CHAPTER 4:
Save Money 49

CHAPTER 5:
Drink More Water 59

CHAPTER 6:
Spend More Quality Time with Family 67

CHAPTER 7:
Tend to Your Mental Health 79

CHAPTER 8:
Take Your Vitamins and Medicines as Prescribed 91

CHAPTER 9:
Relax, Smile, and Be Merry 103

CHAPTER 10:
Get an Annual Physical 109

CHAPTER 11:
Treat Your Body as a Temple 119

CHAPTER 12:
Don't Stress Over Things You Can't Control 127

Conclusion 141

Thank You 143

Sources 147

About the Author 149

Introduction

Experience is a great teacher and renders one an expert, with the ability to pass on their knowledge to others and help them along their journey. My father always said, "Buy your experiences second hand, it won't cost you as much." I've learned that to be true. Because of my life experiences, my goal is to help others like me (Christians, busy individuals, family supporters, ministers) avoid some of the money lost, time spent, heartache, and "bumps in the road," on this journey to achieving health and wellness.

I was raised in a loving home with two wonderful parents, who were full-time pastors and also worked other full-time careers while managing the home and working in the community. My parents were always on the go, always helping, and often neglecting their own health to minister to others. It was watching them in action, always in overdrive, eventually driving themselves toward unhealthy, unfulfilled existences that encouraged me to write this book. I wanted to help them, myself, and others like us to find abundant life. Thankfully, they were able to push pause before driving themselves into early graves and learn how to say yes to themselves, making changes to better their situation and be genuinely happy.

I had the experience most Pastor's Kids (PKs) lived: growing up in church, always in the public eye, working in all ministries and departments at the church, and learning the lies of the Messiah Trap early: If I don't do it, it won't get done, and everyone else's needs come before my own. I was the proverbial first-born child: the high achiever, the kid who excelled at everything (music, sports, academics, the socialite), the kid who learned to show that everything was perfect, even if it wasn't. I announced at 4-years-old that I would be a doctor and deliver babies, and my parents, who are big supporters of education, helped me to hone in on this dream by buying me medical books and enrolling me in pre-med programs throughout my childhood and adolescence. My parents sent me to Oral Roberts University, a Christian college, where I obtained three degrees: a bachelor's degree in Pre-med Psychology, a master's degree in Marriage and Family Therapy, and another master's degree in Christian Counseling. After working as a therapist for a few years, I went on to medical school to reach my ultimate goal of becoming a physician. Along the way, I experienced ups and downs with my own health and didn't always do things to optimize wellness. After graduating from medical school and residency training, I should have been at the prime of my life. Instead, I found myself in a large amount of debt, depressed, and morbidly obese, weighing over 350 pounds. One morning during my quiet time, I read Luke 4:23, and it resonated with me, saying "Physician, heal thyself!" I knew I had to make some changes. I set off on a journey to improve my health in totality, transforming my habits and changing my body, mind, spirit, and finances. What I learned on my transformation I decided to write down, so that I can help you and others who are struggling with their health, to change, and prosper and be in health, even as their souls prosper (3 John 1:2 KJV).

I know the value of improving health firsthand, as I have overcome depression and career burnout. I have been able to lose over 125 pounds, live optimistically despite having chronic medical conditions that would discourage most people, and work with ministers and congregations, witnessing the outcomes of changing habits and mindsets to lead to healthier lives. I have helped Pastors lose weight, which improved their energy and stamina, helping them preach better and to overcome stress and depression. I also helped them to become aware of their financial state and learn to save money. I am honored that I work in a career that embodies Christ, who was known as the Great Physician, Jehovah Rapha, and the Balm in Gilead. God created the body and takes great pride in His creation. It hurts Him to see His creation hurting and sick, so He sent Jesus to heal mankind. Isaiah 53: 4-5 (NIV) tells us, "Surely he took up our pain and bore our suffering, yet we considered him punished by God, stricken by him, and afflicted. But he was pierced for our transgressions, he was crushed for our iniquities; the punishment that brought us peace was on him, and by his wounds we are healed." Many of the parables in the New Testament were about healing: Timothy had a sour stomach and had to learn the medicinal effects of wine. Peter's mother-in-law was sick with fever. One woman had a problem with a prolonged heavy menstrual cycle. Many people were blind, deaf, or unable to walk. There is even a story of a man dealing with rage and uncontrollable thoughts and actions. God knows what His creation needs and just as He sent His Son Jesus and the disciples to heal those in Bible days, He has equipped individuals now, such as pastors, counselors, and doctors, to be a part of the healing ministry. My ministry is not only through song during praise and worship or playing the keyboard. It is daily, when I help people normalize their blood pressure, help clients lose weight and overcome depression and anxiety, help pastors recognize life-threatening illnesses like heart disease or mini-strokes, and help readers achieve divine healing. Jesus invoked multiple methods to bring healing to the masses. Sometimes it was through laying hands; sometimes He used saliva and mud; sometimes He just spoke a word, and sometimes He even had to heal the same person more than once. The bottom line is that God wanted His people to be healthy by any means necessary.

Throughout this book, you will learn the practical steps that I've used to change the lives of my patients, clients, and even myself. The "secrets" I discuss in this book are actually well-known facts to improving health, but I prefer to call them secrets because everyone may not know them, and people who know about them may not know how to implement them in their everyday lives. The scriptures at the end of each chapter should be used as a reference for further Biblical meaning, and as a guide to study the Bible to see what God says in His word about each secret. Proverbs 4:20-22 (ESV) tells us, *"My son, be attentive to my words; incline your ear to my sayings. Let them not escape from your sight; keep them within your heart. For they are life to those who find them, and healing to all their flesh."* Use the "Practice What You Preach" section at the end of each chapter to implement some of the steps I discuss, and as a guide to changing your actions to improve your life. By using the secrets to positively transform your life, you will be able to embrace God's will for your life and walk in complete healing as He intended. In Exodus 15:26 MSG, "God said, *'If you listen, listen obediently to how I tell you to live in my presence, obeying my commandments and keeping all my laws, then I won't strike you with all the diseases that I inflicted on the Egyptians; I am God your healer.'"*

Revisit the devotional and Practice What You Preach sections at least bi-monthly to track your progress and gain a refresher on the topics. As you implement these secrets in your everyday life, you will see a positive difference in your attitude, body structure, energy levels, spirituality, and finances.

"Nevertheless, I will bring health and healing to it; I will heal my people and will let them enjoy abundant peace and security."

Jeremiah 33:6 NIV

1

Meditate Daily

"This Book of the Law shall not depart from your mouth, but you shall meditate in it day and night, that you may observe to do according to all that is written in it. For then you will make your way prosperous, and then you will have good success."

Joshua 1:8 NKJV

Picture, if you will, the daily life of a busy Family Medicine Physician. I wake up, get myself and the kids ready, take the kids to school while listening to their singing and playing, and sometimes fighting, then make the drive in to work. At work, I see 20-25 patients per day, in 15-30 minute time slots. Those slots often aren't long enough, so I fall behind, which is frustrating for the other patients and for me. I deal with patients who are ill, dying, scared, and sometimes angry. They bring me their problems, coughing and sneezing in the room, covering me with their germs. They cry on my shoulder, try to prove they are smarter than me with their Google searches, and sometimes cuss at me because they're mad at their failing health or at the insurance company for not authorizing the test or medication they wanted. Occasionally, but rarely, some say thank you. It's not uncommon to have to stay at work past the time that the clinic doors actually close, trying to complete charts and sign off on paperwork, and argue with the insurance companies on behalf of patients. I'm rarely home at a decent hour. Then I go home to make dinner, help the kids with their homework, clean up, and try to spend some time with my husband before finally falling into bed, exhausted and often dreading having to get up and do it all again the next day. I had to develop a coping mechanism.

With a schedule this demanding, I had to figure out how to locate some peace and quiet so I could energize myself. I started by taking the 20 minutes of quiet time in the car after dropping off the kids, to turn off the morning radio show, and either drive in silence or with some calming peaceful music. I made a playlist called Morning Smile to listen to, and help me clear my thoughts and prepare for what could be a hectic day. You know what I found by doing that? I found that the days didn't seem as long, and I was able to better handle some of the stressful situations. I also began taking a minute after seeing a difficult or angry patient, to take a walk around the parking lot or down the street so I could pray, sing, listen to a happy song, or sometimes just scream to the atmosphere, instead of taking my frustrations out on the next patient or my staff. I found that locating that quiet place in my spirit and mind helped to keep me grounded. I now incorporate quiet meditation into my day as a routine, and I have seen the difference it makes.

Meditation is defined as the practice of engaging in thought, reflection, or contemplation; engaging in quiescent spiritual introspection. It helps to quiet the mind and reset thoughts and ideas. There benefits to meditation are that it reduces stress, improves blood flow and cardiovascular health, clears the mind and allows for refocusing, increases happiness, and slows the aging process. Meditation does not require chanting "Om," as most people imagine when they think of meditation done by Buddhist monks, and it can be done by anyone regardless of religion or age.

I've seen the effects of stress, anger, and hurt in people, especially those who do not meditate, and it can affect them mentally and physically. People who neglect self-care often have problems with fatigue, back and neck pain, stomach issues like Irritable Bowel Syndrome (IBS), and interpersonal problems with their family and friends. People often feel like the weight of the world is on their shoulders and instead of offloading that weight, they carry their depression, anxiety and insomnia around with them. Hebrews 12:1 (NIV) says, "let us throw off everything that hinders and the sin that so easily entangles," and this can be done through meditation.

Many people designate an area of their home to set the atmosphere for meditation and reflection, as it is best to practice meditation in a quiet place of solitude. It is important to have a set place or routine to follow for meditation. By incorporating this routine, your body is trained to recognize that you are in a safe place and can relax, which is crucial for effective meditation. If you are physically or mentally uneasy, your body will go into fight- or-flight mode, making relaxation and meditation non-existent or ineffective. There are many ways to create a space for meditation. I have seen people make prayer closets or set off a corner of a room with pillows and comfortable seating. Some choose rooms with nice lighting or a great view, or decorate rooms specifically for meditation. Décor can include inspirational pictures or posters, special lighting fixtures and lamps with a dimmer to control the atmosphere, sculptures or figures that invoke peace or hope, oil and aroma diffusers, and sometimes a sound system to play quiet music. I personally changed a room in my home to my "happy place," complete with nice lighting, temperature control for my comfort, a sound system, an aroma diffuser, comfortable seating, and pictures that calm me. I have vowed to not do any work in the room and no arguing or loud voices are allowed, to ensure a tranquil, happy atmosphere. Since building my Happy Place, I have made it a point to use it frequently. It has helped me unwind, center myself, and decrease stress levels.

During meditation, you can pray, read scripture, listen to quiet music, do yoga, or any activity that can be done with minimal effort or thinking. Some also exercise or stretch during meditation. I recommend choosing a topic or theme and focusing on that choice for your meditation session. You can think of how that topic/subject can help you currently or in the future, and what you need to do to implement it more often. Many people use a meditation guide or devotional book to help select their topics and guide their mindset during meditation. There are a myriad of books and devotional meditation plans on apps and devices that are available to help individuals with meditation. The books and plans guide the reader to different areas that can be explored and then give practical suggestions on how to use the information received from the introspection. Other meditation plans focus on scriptures and can show the reader how to read the Bible with understanding.

Meditation doesn't have to be a long period. Sometimes 10-15 minutes is all that is necessary. It is not about the quantity of time spent in meditation; it is about the quality of centering yourself and resetting your energy through meditation that makes it effective. Many people meditate during a commute to or from work, which can help them prepare for the day or decompress before they get home, so that they can keep work separate from their home life. People can also meditate while getting ready in the morning, sometimes through exercise, or eating a hearty breakfast while drinking a cup of coffee. Whenever you can find 5-10 minutes, meditate and see how much clearer and focused you'll be for the rest of the day.

Meditation is great for clearing the mind and gives the ability to start fresh with a clean slate. Because we in western society have so much going on constantly with phones, computers, televisions, busy-work, multiple jobs, and the hustle and bustle of life in general, we need to have dedicated quiet time. Quiet time does not mean there shouldn't be any music or noise, but the noise needs to be white noise, like quiet calming music to help keep the mind clear and relaxed. If your mind begins to cloud with thoughts of business or day planning, reset and start quieting the mind again. It is very common for the mind to wander during quiet time, but be sure to think of positive things. If negativity comes to mind, immediately stop that thought and focus on positive ideas. It is useful to have a list of positive subjects to focus on in case you need some mental guidance. Philippians 4:8 (ASV) says to think on things that are true, honorable, right, pure, lovely, and of good report. Let this be a guide on what to focus on during meditation.

Meditate Day and Night

"I will meditate on Your precepts and regard Your ways. I shall delight in Your statutes; I shall not forget Your word."

Psalm 119:15-16 NASB

"I remember the days of old; I meditate on all Your doings; I muse on the work of Your hands."

Psalm 143:5 NASB

"Consider what I say, for the Lord will give you understanding in everything."

2 Timothy 2:7 NASB

Practice What You Preach

List 3 quiet places you can meditate

List 3 ways you can clear your mind before meditation.

List 3 of your favorite scriptures or inspirational quotes to meditate on.

List 3 of your favorite songs (usually without words or minimal lyrics) to meditate to.

2

Eat More Fruits and Vegetables

But Daniel purposed in his heart that he would not defile himself with the portion of the king's delicacies, nor with the wine which he drank; therefore he requested of the chief of the eunuchs that he might not defile himself. And the chief of the eunuchs said to Daniel, "I fear my lord the king, who has appointed your food and drink. For why should he see your faces looking worse than the young men who are your age? Then you would endanger my head before the king." So Daniel said to the steward whom the chief of the eunuchs had set over Daniel, Hananiah, Mishael, and Azariah, "Please test your servants for ten days, and let them give us vegetables to eat and water to drink. Then let our appearance be examined before you, and the appearance of the young men who eat the portion of the king's delicacies; and as you see fit, so deal with your servants." So he consented with them in this matter, and tested them ten days. And at the end of ten days their features appeared better and fatter in flesh than all the young men who ate the portion of the king's delicacies.

Daniel 1:8-15 NKJV

The story of Daniel and the Hebrew boys is not just a Biblical story or fable. I have done a Daniel Fast, where I and other members in my accountability tram had only fruit, vegetables, and water for 21 days. We lost weight, gained muscle, slept better, our skin was clearer, our minds were clearer. We felt better and had more energy. Many personal trainers and dieticians encourage eating less meat, dairy, and animal based products to improve health.

Despite an increasing number of healthy-living trends, people in modern western society do not eat enough fruits and vegetables. Older generations were typically healthier because they cultivated the land and ate the fruits of their labor. Children often do not eat enough fruits and vegetables because their parents don't model that healthy behavior, and we are now seeing an increase in the numbers of children with obesity, elevated cholesterol, and high blood sugar (symptoms of metabolic syndrome). I get it. I know that when you are already tired after a long day, it's quicker and easier to cook boxed meals. But those meals come at a price. They are chocked full of preservatives and artificial flavors, and do not involve much fresh produce. I'm reminded of the saying: you can have it fast, have it cheap, or have it good, but you can only get two. If it's fast and good, it's not cheap. If it's fast and cheap, it's not good. If it's good and cheap, it's not fast. The same holds true for food. If it's fast and cheap, like that microwave TV dinner, it's not good for you. If it's good and cheap, like the foods that are grown in the garden, it's not fast (we all know it takes some time for food to be grown in a garden).

In today's microwave society, we eat more artificial, processed foods that are quick to heat up and can be stored longer due to preservatives. Processed foods may be cheaper at times, but reasonably priced produce can be found at farmers markets or flea markets. Although those foods will have to be purchased weekly, losing the benefit of convenience, you gain longevity and better health by eating fresh. If you compare a box of pasta to fresh fruit, the shelf lives are vastly different. Fresh fruit and vegetables last only 3-5 days where processed foods can last months. Healthy food is better for digestive health, as it does not contain preservatives and can be processed quickly to the necessary nutrients for cell growth. It's "shelf-life" is short by design because it's natural, and the human body is healthier when it is fed natural foods. Packaged, canned, or processed foods contain artificial preservatives and sodium which can elevate blood pressure and damage the kidneys, heart, and brain. In grocery stores, the fresh fruit and vegetables are on the outer aisles while the processed foods are in the center aisles. Aim to shop in the outer aisles more for a balanced, healthier diet.

A lot of children (and even some adults) think vegetables taste nasty, so they don't try to incorporate them into their daily meals. They've never had asparagus flavored with garlic and Italian seasoning, or sweet potatoes without covering them in molasses and butter. The first step in accepting more fruits and vegetables is to be open to trying new things. Once you open your mind to the idea of trying new fruits and vegetables, the next step is finding good spices for seasoning, and good recipes for preparing those foods. Finally, the last step in eating more fruits and vegetables is to taste and see that it is good, and eat more of it!

There are multiple benefits to eating more fruit and vegetables. Diets that contain fruits and vegetables provide vitamins and minerals that are important for good health. Studies have shown that fruits and vegetables can reduce the risk of cancer, improve health and vitality, heal and build up the body from a cellular level, and improve and prevent chronic disease. Multiple medical boards and healthy lifestyle programs agree that increasing fruit and vegetables in your diet help you by increasing fiber intake that keep your digestive system regular, improving circulation so that oxygen and antibodies can flow freely through the body. This prevents cardiovascular disease and assists with weight loss. Fruits and vegetables are a fun to eat, taste great, are nutritious, can be grown in your own backyard, and can be consumed in any form: fresh, frozen, canned, dried, puréed, or blended. Fruit and vegetables add color and texture to your plate which keeps your meals new and exciting!

Many of you reading this book are busy in the ministry of helping others, whether you are a teacher, counselor, parent, pastor, or entrepreneur. When you are giving your time and effort, often physically and mentally, your body needs specific nutrients from fruit and vegetables to continue to function optimally. The Huffington Post article *Benefits Of fruits and Vegetables* by Dr. Lisa Young, published on July 12, 2012 gives a comprehensive list of different fruits and vegetables and their benefits. I have listed some of that list below:

Green leafy vegetables like broccoli, kale, collards, cabbage, and cauliflower have antioxidant properties which can protect the body from breakdown and from harmful viruses and illness. Broccoli is full of vitamin C, the mineral calcium, fiber, and vitamin A that can fight cancer and improve the immune system. These green leafy vegetables also assist in moving the bowels and preventing bloating, stomach aches, and constipation.

Carrots are a good source of fiber, which helps to maintain bowel health, lower blood cholesterol, and aid in weight maintenance. The orange pigment found in carrots and other deep orange foods such as sweet potatoes, pumpkin, butternut squash, papaya, and cantaloupe is beta-carotene which helps to maintain healthy eyes, support your immune system, keep your skin healthy, and protect against certain cancers.

Spinach contains the minerals iron and potassium, as well as vitamins A, K, C, and the B-vitamin folate. Spinach may boost your immune system and may be preventative against certain cancers.

Sweet Potatoes are rich in beta-carotene and are also full of fiber, vitamin B6, folate, vitamin C, and potassium. They are especially nutritious when eaten with the skin on, and contrary to a popular dieting myth, they are not fattening!

Beets contain healthy doses of iron, the B-vitamin folate, and fiber. Red beets offer betacyanin, a plant pigment that may protect against colon cancer, which is high in occurrence in African American and Hispanic men age 50 and over.

Citrus fruits, including oranges and grapefruits, provide a significant source of vitamin C, folate, antioxidants, and potassium, as well as fiber. This is essential for those in careers where they are around other people, as this helps strengthen the immune system and fight against germs and infections. .

Avocados are rich in heart-healthy monounsaturated fats, which may help raise levels of HDL (good cholesterol) while lowering LDL (bad cholesterol). They are also high in the antioxidant vitamin E.

Grapes may reduce the risk of blood clots, lower LDL, and prevent damage to the heart's blood vessels, aiding in the maintenance of healthy blood pressure. Antioxidants in grapes, called flavonoids, may even increase HDL cholesterol, while the skins of red grapes may interfere with cancer development. Eating the whole fruit instead of consuming the juice contains the added benefit of fiber.

There are a myriad of other fruits and vegetables, all of which are good for you and taste great. The goal should be 2-3 servings of fruit or vegetables (preferably green leafy vegetables) per meal each day. Don't forget that fruit and vegetables also count as a great healthy snack! My motto is: if it's grown from a plant, eat it. If it's grown in a plant (factory), don't!

Meditate Day and Night

*"Whether, then, you eat or drink or whatever you do,
do all to the glory of God."*

1 Corinthians 10:31 NASB

*"And God said, 'Behold, I have given you every plant
yielding seed that is on the face of all the earth, and every
tree with seed in its fruit. You shall have them for food."*

Genesis 1:29 ESV

*"And on the banks, on both sides of the river,
there will grow all kinds of trees for food. Their leave
will not wither, nor their fruit fail, but they will bear fresh
fruit every month, because the water for them flows
from the sanctuary. Their fruit will be for food,
and their leaves for healing."*

Ezekiel 47:12 ESV

Practice What You Preach

List your favorite fruits and vegetables.

List 3 different ways to prepare your favorite fruits or vegetables.

Set a challenge to eat only fruits vegetables and water for 7-10 days. List your starting weight and how you feel each day, then your ending weight. Did you see any improvement in weight, energy, clarity, skin, etc.?

Starting Weight: _____   Ending Weight _____

Day 1 Food Log:

_____

_____

Day 1 Feelings:

_____

_____

_____

_____

Day 2 Food Log:

_____

_____

Day 2 Feelings:

Day 3 Food Log:

Day 3 Feelings:

Day 4 Food Log:

Day 4 Feelings:

Day 5 Food Log:

Day 5 Feelings:

Day 6 Food Log:

Day 6 Feelings:

Day 7 Food Log:

Day 7 Feelings:

Day 8 Food Log:

Day 8 Feelings:

Day 9 Food Log:

Day 9 Feelings:

Day 10 Food Log:

Day 10 Feelings:

3

Exercise More

"He gives power to the faint, abundant strength to the weak. Though young men faint and grow weary, and youths stagger and fall, they that hope in the lord will renew their strength, they will soar on eagles' wings; They will run and not grow weary, walk and not grow faint."

Isaiah 40:29-31, NABRE

What is the number one New Year's Resolution? To exercise more! More gym memberships and fitness apps are sold at the end of the year and first few days of the year because people resolve that this is the year they will get healthy. Many regular gym and exercise connoisseurs get a bit annoyed at the beginning of the year because their once empty gym is full of new customers limiting the equipment and filling the exercise space. Fortunately for the gym regulars, but unfortunately for the New Year Resolvers and new fitness seekers, most of the gym newbies wean themselves out by the third or fourth week of January once the newness of the New Year fades away and regular life routines take over, pushing exercise to the back burner.

Most people are aware of the benefits of exercise because it is discussed and stressed in so many different arenas like the doctor's office, in the media, and at school with physical education. Even religion, the Bible, and church stress the importance of exercise with over 75 scriptures in the Holy Bible discussing physical exercise and fitness. Churches have been implementing exercise and physical fitness into their worship experiences by having Move Sunday or Fitness Worship, where the members wear sweats or workout clothes, and do workout routines during Praise and Worship to encourage movement. One Pastor, who I coached through exercise and healthy living, lost over 60 pounds and was able to preach longer without getting winded, was able to do more community work without being as tired, and had an overall improvement in his health resulting in getting off many of his medications and requiring less doctor's visits. Benefits such as increasing cardiovascular output and strength, decreasing stress by releasing natural endorphins, improving flexibility, lowering the risk of type-2 diabetes, high blood pressure, and high cholesterol, and improving appearance and self-esteem by helping with weight loss are often common knowledge, but most people struggle with knowing how to exercise properly, and how to implement exercise into their already busy routines.

I recommend getting a trainer to show you how to effectively strength train and implement your workout into your busy schedule. The benefit of having a trainer, even if it is just for a few sessions, is to show you things like how to activate and work different muscle groups, and the antagonist muscles that are also strengthened with each exercise. The trainer can show you proper techniques like positioning and stance that help isolate the specific muscle group you are working on, and how to have a more effective workout. Some people may object to having a trainer because they may feel embarrassed by their fitness level (or lack thereof), but trainers are aware that you likely don't know what you are doing and they are sensitive to this and have dealt with others just like you. Other reasons people object to trainers is modesty or concern for having a trainer of the opposite sex, but in this day and age, you can find trainers of all genders, ages, and walks of life; there is a trainer for everyone, whatever will make you feel comfortable. Another excuse people use for not getting a trainer is cost, but getting a trainer to show you how to work out correctly and safely can save you time, effort, and even money because if you were to injure yourself doing an exercise incorrectly, it would cost a lot more to get treatment for the injury.

Your trainer will teach you that exercise can and should be challenging. Exercise done effectively should cause you to break a sweat and be winded, but still able to carry on a conversation. I've found that exercise gives me a boost when

I've had a long day or if I'm under a lot of stress. I often use my workout to take out my frustrations. For example, a good kickboxing or punching the boxing bag routine is especially helpful after dealing with difficult people or not having a good day. I know that having a long or busy day can often be the excuse people use to forego a workout, but these are the times that more effort should be given to exercising to help lower stress and cortisol levels, and stretch the muscles where stress hormones may be accumulating, resulting in spasms and myalgias (muscle pains).

Exercise should be fun and enjoyable, giving reason to want to continue long-term. Exercise can be fun by doing a form of exercise like a dance class or trampoline class. I've seen exercises that incorporated certain types of music and rhythmic moving while on exercise bikes or balls. Exercise also becomes fun when you do it with a friend or family member who can laugh with, and in some cases, at you! The more fun and exciting a class is, the more people want to return and bring guests. I've seen water aerobics, Zumba classes, cross fit courses, and trampoline classes, where the entire class was laughing and having a great time, and that made me want to try the class for myself to see what all the hype was!

There are different types of exercise: strength training, stretching, and cardiovascular training. All of them are important depending on the expected outcome. Cardiovascular exercise helps burn fat and increase stamina. Stretching increases flexibility and muscle tone, and strength training builds muscle. All forms of exercise improve blood flow so you can't go wrong with any of the types. Each individual needs to assess their starting fitness level before engaging in an exercise program and have clearly defined goals that can be modified if needed during the workout time. Keep in mind that one workout plan does not fit all, and you should know this before joining group classes.

Cardiovascular training and exercise occurs when the activity causes the heart rate to go up and is maintained at a level that makes the heart rate, blood pressure, and cardiac motility and strength go up. The heart is a muscle and has to be trained and kept healthy through exercise and maintaining good blood flow to the coronary arteries (the arteries bring blood to the heart). When the heart is not healthy, it can result in heart failure and coronary artery disease, which can lead to heart attacks, cardiac muscle damage and cell death. Walking, bike riding, aerobics classes, Zumba, swimming, elliptical machines, trampoline classes, running, and kickboxing are all examples of cardiovascular exercise.

Strength training is another form of exercise that is also essential to increasing muscle mass to help sculpt the body and burn fat. This form of exercise is best for people looking to tone muscles, tighten skin, increase muscle size and appearance, and burn fat faster. A balance of cardiovascular exercise and strength training is best to improve health, as the increased blood flow from both forms will help increase oxygenation to the tissues. Fat will be burned faster when the two are done together. Strength training can be done in a gym with a trainer or on your own, but it can even be done at home. Using hand held weights, even as small as 1 to 2 pounds, can help increase muscle mass and strength. Repetition is as important as the weight of the objects you are lifting, and sometimes doing more repetitions with lower weights can result in more muscle mass without as much damage to the muscle fibers. If you are exercising at home, you can get small hand held weights, or use objects around the house like cans of food, stretchy bands, or even a gallon of milk. Strength training helps to tone the muscles that are revealed as you lose fat and weight. Muscle training like sit-ups is helpful, but if there is a layer of fat around the muscle, it will be difficult to see the increased mass of the muscles. For this reason, it is good to incorporate both cardiovascular exercise to help burn the fat and strength training to tone the muscles. Strength training also helps to burn fat, so the two should be done in conjunction with each other.

Also included, but sometimes forgotten in the exercise regiment, is stretching. Stretching helps to elongate and stretch muscle fibers which help with elasticity, flexibility and in the long-term, strength, by improving muscle tone. There are different kinds of stretching: active, passive, dynamic, and static. All should be done until a safe, gentle pulling sensation is achieved, but should not hurt or be too uncomfortable.

Tai-Chi and Yoga are great forms of exercise that incorporate stretching. After stretching, toxins can be released from the spasms and knots that build up in the muscles. It is best to drink a lot of water, and eat some protein after stretching and exercising to help the body regenerate the muscle tissue and flush the toxins that we're released.

Everyone, of all ages, both genders, and any walk of life should exercise. I know that being busy with life as a parent, entrepreneur, student, or employee can put major constraints on your time. Believe me, as a wife, mother, employee, business owner, minister, radio and television personality, sorority member, friend, and active community member, I know firsthand that time to exercise can often be pushed to the back burner. However, I understand the importance of exercise, and I know that I feel much better physically and mentally after I exercise. I have started combining some of my tasks into my exercise routine to optimize my time. Sometimes I exercise with my kids by going to the park and walking the track while they ride their bikes, or we play a video game that requires movement together. I can go to a fun exercise class with my family and friends or play tennis with my husband, fulfilling quality time with loved ones and exercise. I can also read or answer emails while on an exercise machine like the elliptical machine or recumbent bike. Finding the time to exercise can be challenging, but it can be done! I know because I have been doing it for years, and it has helped me shed over one hundred pounds!

If you are aiming for weight loss, you need 30-45 minutes of cardiovascular exercise, 5-6 days a week to lose more calories than you consume. If you are looking for weight maintenance, you need 30 minutes, 3-4 days per week, which is typically the same amount of calories lost that the typical person takes in on a weekly basis. If you burn the same amount of calories that you consume, you will stay the same weight. Exercise can be done with a group, which is great for accountability and support, or alone which is great for clearing the mind and a form of meditation.

Before beginning an exercise program, you should check with your doctor to ensure your body is healthy enough for the exercise program and type that you choose. Even if you cannot do one type of exercise, as in the case of an injury, your doctor can give you other exercises that can be done safely and effectively to achieve the increased heart rate and cardiovascular output to help improve your health. I have patients who cannot handle load bearing exercise due to joint injuries, or foot injuries/conditions. For those patients, I prescribe an exercise plan that involves weightless water aerobics, or the use of a table bike or a recumbent bike, which still enables cardiovascular increase without the weight bearing, which can worsen their injury or condition.

Before starting an exercise plan, set goals so you can have something to work toward and remember why you are working out. I encourage people to write out their goals, or hang up the outfit they are trying to fit into as motivation and encouragement to continue their exercise efforts. My personal goal for working out was to increase my stamina so I wouldn't be out of breath when I went up a flight of stairs. I've seen people use their children or grandchildren for motivation so that they can run around and play with them without getting tired and so that they can be around to see them grow up and have families of their own. Be sure to set are small, achievable goals. If you set too large a goal, it is easy to get discouraged if the goal is not reached. For example: While the goal to lose 100 pounds is feasible over a significant amount of time, it can be daunting; if after a month of exercising, you only lose 7 or 8 pounds, you may become discouraged, decreasing your motivation, which leads to quitting. However, if you set an attainable goal of 10 pounds per month, that can be achieved through hard work and dedication. Once you lose the first 10 pounds, you are likely to maintain the motivation to keep going, losing another 10, and another 10. Before you know it, a 10-pound weight loss goal turns into to 100 pounds lost in about a year!

A good workout will be challenging and can even be hard at times. Using a trainer can help to motivate and push you toward your goals, and holds you accountable so that you don't give up. If you cannot afford a trainer, find an accountability partner who can also motivate you to keep going. I once had an accountability partner who would call me when I didn't feel like exercising, and come over to my house to bother me until I put on my workout clothes and began my workout. I would do the same for her. Studies have shown that weight loss and exercise are best maintained in a group setting with accountability. Be sure to surround yourself with people who will encourage you, help you to reach your goals, and even work with you toward achieving those goals.

Meditate Day and Night

"Do you not know that in a race all the runners run [their very best to win], but only one receives the prize? Run [your race] in such a way that you may seize the prize and make it yours! Now every athlete who [goes into training and] competes in the games is disciplined and exercises self-control in all things. They do it to win a crown that withers, but we [do it to receive] an imperishable [crown that cannot wither]. Therefore I do not run without a definite goal; I do not flail around like one beating the air [just shadow boxing]. But [like a boxer] I strictly discipline my body and make it my slave, so that, after I have preached [the gospel] to others, I myself will not somehow be disqualified [as unfit for service]."

1 Corinthians 9:24-27 AMP

"She girds herself with strength; she exerts her arms with vigor."

Proverbs 31:17 NABRE

"A wise man is fully of strength, and a man of knowledge enhances his might."

Proverbs 24:5 ESV

"I have completed well; I have finished the race; I have kept the faith."

2 Timothy 4:7 USCCB

Practice What You Preach

List your three accountability partners and set group goals (example: exercise 3 days a week together; call each other 15 minutes before the scheduled workout time; join a program like MyFitnessPal or try a Fitbit challenge, etc.).

_____

_____

_____

Write an exercise schedule. Try to do something a bit different each day to work different muscles. Don't forget to incorporate a rest day! Do at least 30 minutes of exercise each day. For example: Day1- walk for 30minutes, Day 2- lower body strength training, Day 3- bike for 30 minutes, Day 4-upper body strength training, Day 5- exercise class like Zumba or cross training, Day 6- abs and gluts (butt) workout, Day 7-rest

Day 1: _____

Day 2: _____

Day 3: _____

Day 4: _____

Day 5: _____

Day 6: _____

Day 7: _____

Write out your exercise goals and the lifestyle changes you will use to meet and exceed those goals. For example: 25-pound weight loss, increase stamina, walk up a set of stairs without becoming winded, increase flexibility, etc.

Write out your current weight and measurements, and update the numbers every 2-4 weeks.

	Current	2 weeks	4 weeks	6 weeks	8 weeks	2 weeks
Weight						
Neck						
Chest						
Biceps						
Forearms						
Waist						
Hips						
Thighs						
Calves						
% Body Fat						

4

Save Money

"On the first day of every week, each of you should set aside a sum of money in keeping with your income, saving it up, so that when I come no collections will have to be made."

1 Corinthians 16:2 NIV

When discussing whole-man health, it is important to include all parts of man: mind, body, and spirit. One often neglected portion of the makeup of man is how he deals with finances, as this can affect all three parts. Money affects the body by providing or losing the ability to feed, clothe, cover (with housing), and engage the body in self-care. Money affects the mind and spirit by providing a sense of or lack of security, which can cause joy or satisfaction when money is in excess, and fear, worry, depression, and anger when money is at a deficit. Money and possessions are the second most referenced topic in the Bible, where money is mentioned over 800 times. Grandich, author of *Confessions of A Wall Street Whiz Kid*, states that the answers to all sorts of money issues can be found in the Bible, and that is where he gets his financial guidance.

Examples of issues discussed in the bible include lending and borrowing, investing and turning a profit, and even preparation for emergencies and rainy days. Ecclesiastes 11:2 (NIV) says *"Invest in seven ventures, yes in eight; you do not know what disaster may come upon the land,"* encouraging us to e save money and have a safety net for emergencies and for the future. I know that it can be difficult to set aside and save money, as there are often more bills and problems per month than there is paycheck, but small steps can be used to add up to a substantial savings. By saving small amounts, such as spare change or a few dollars per week, it can add up to large amounts over time. Eliminate unnecessary bills like automatic payments for things that are not used, like apps or games, to save a few dollars each month. Cutting back on cell phone bills or cable packages is another way to save a few dollars. Take the money saved and invest it in a mutual fund, savings account, CD or other investment option. Most financial planners recommend having 3 months' salary set aside for incidentals and emergencies, on top of a savings account and retirement fund. This 3 months' salary does not have to be set aside all at once. Small increments can eventually grow to 3 months' salary in a savings account that can be accessed without penalty, but should only be used in case of emergency. You should write what constitutes an emergency: car breaking down, home repairs, illness, etc., and only use the emergency fund for true emergencies. Once monies are built up, you can find other ways to lower payments such as picking an insurance plan with a higher deductible but lower monthly premium, which will save you money over time.

The amount of savings varies for each individual but a good starting goal is to save 10-15 percent of your salary. People allocate funds in different ways. Some set aside 10 percent for savings, 10 percent for tithes/donations, 60 percent for bills, and 20 percent for self-care. The best advice I ever heard about saving money was from my college professor, who suggested saving $50 per paycheck starting at age 18, and depositing the savings into a mutual fund. Following that advice, the mutual fund would be worth over one million dollars by age 40. Most people don't plan on working until they die, so it is necessary to start a savings or retirement fund as early as possible. Many people put off savings accounts and retirement funds assuming that they will have time to do it later. Unfortunately, we never know when an emergency can occur, and the possibility of disability or even death can occur any time. Most people don't anticipate having a car accident, but we all pay for car insurance despite having claims or not. We should look at savings account funds in the same manner. Hopefully we never have to use it, but better to have it and not need it, than need it and not have it. The other advantage of starting a retirement fund earlier is that you can allocate smaller amounts for a longer time, rather than to being forced to put in large amounts as you get closer to retirement age. There are also tax breaks and benefits available for contributing funds to retirement accounts.

Many companies offer 401K or 403B programs where the employer matches a percentage of the funds you put in to the account. Employer contributions stay in the account as long as you work for the company, or until you become vested (employees must remain employed for a certain amount of time to keep the money they contributed to the account). This is a great way to gain additional retirement funds, so be sure to ask about this benefit when you are applying for jobs, or in a salary negotiation process.

It may be wise to seek the assistance of an accountant or tax specialist to help explain and navigate your finances. Having a financial planner is also great so that you know exactly how to diversify or spread your money, which allows your initial investment to make money for you. Many financial planners do not charge for the initial consultation to analyze your current budget to help you set goals and make a plan. It may seem daunting to see all of these finance specialists at once, or to even think of how to go from managing your own money to needing to see a specialist, but I would recommend starting with the financial planner. They can tell you if any other specialists are needed for your specific financial situation.

Before you go in to see your financial planner, it is best to already have goals and an idea of where you want to see your money in the future. You should write out your financial goals for the month, year, 5 years, 10 years, 25 years, and into retirement so that you know how you will need to save to achieve these goals. Every person's plan will be different based on the desired outcome; not everyone wants to have a five-bedroom house with two cars, a boat, and land. Some people want to spend money on travel; some are happy in a small cottage with one car, while others want a luxurious lifestyle. Whatever your goals, your financial planner will review future plans and show you how to budget to attain those goals. Once you meet with the planner, they will suggest a schedule to follow-up to review your goals, and how you have been doing with the savings plan they helped you implement. This should be revisited at least annually, or if there are any changes to your financial status (change in career or job status, change in family size, major change in bills, etc.). Your planner will educate you on how the stock market works, and how to invest your money. When you do invest your money, the advisor will likely teach you how to diversify the holdings; this means that you spread your money into different places which lowers your risk of losing all of your investment if the market crashes or money is lost in one venture.

Saving money ensures a safety net for your future and leaves something to pass on to your children and grandchildren. Some of the soundest advice I ever received was to live life today like no one else does so that tomorrow, you can live life like no one else can. This translates to sacrificing some of the luxuries of living now, so that later on you can enjoy the fruits of your labor and not work until the day you die.

Saving for a financially sound future makes it even more necessary to surround yourself with likeminded people. If you want to own multiple houses, be in real estate, have money in multiple accounts or even the stock market, acquaint yourself with people who are living that lifestyle, and learn from them. Be sure to plan ahead. Even the Bible shows us that only a fool does not plan. I love the old saying that says Fail to plan and you plan to fail.

Meditate Day and Night

"So the king commanded, and they made a chest, and set it without at the gate of the house of Jehovah. And they made a proclamation through Judah and Jerusalem, to bring in for Jehovah the tax that Moses the servant of God laid upon Israel in the wilderness. And all the princes and all the people rejoiced, and brought in, and cast into the chest, until they had made an end. And it was so, that, at what time the chest was brought unto the king's officers by the hand of the Levites, and when they saw that there was much money, the king's scribe and the chief priest's officer came and emptied the chest, and took it, and carried it to its place again. Thus they did day by day, and gathered money in abundance."

2 Chronicles 24:8-11 ASV

"The prudent see danger and take refuge, but the simple keep going and pay the penalty."

Proverbs 27:12 NIV

"Dishonest money dwindles away, but he who gathers money little by little makes it grow."

Proverbs 13:11 NIV

Practice What You Preach

Write out your monthly budget, including money that will be set aside for savings.

Salary

Mortgage/Rent

Electricity

Water/Sewer/Trash

Phone

Internet

Cable

Car note

Gas

Car insurance

Life insurance

Tithes/charity

Saving

Clothing

Tuition/
Student Loans   _____

Food   _____

Self-Care
(gym membership,
exercise classes,
hair skin and
nail grooming)   _____

Open a mutual fund or savings account. Start small, if necessary, at $5-10 dollars per paycheck. When you can do it affordably, increase the amount by $5 per paycheck until you are up to $25/paycheck which equals $50/month.

List the name of your financial advisor and their contact information. Write out any questions you have so you don't forget to ask. Don't' be afraid to tell them that you don't know things. It is very common to not know what we don't know, but the advisor should be aware of that. You should have great rapport with the advisor and be able to talk with them openly without fear of judgment.

_____

_____

Meet with a financial planner and develop a savings plan. List at least 3 ways you will save money for the future.

How would you like to live in the future? Write out your goals and what it will take to make that a reality.

5

Drink More Water

"And Moses led Israel onward from the Red Sea, and they went out into the wilderness of Shur; and they went three days in the wilderness, and found no water. And when they came to Marah, they could not drink of the waters of Marah, for they were bitter: therefore the name of it was called Marah. And the people murmured against Moses, saying, What shall we drink? And he cried unto Jehovah; And Jehovah showed him a tree, and he cast it into the waters, and the waters were made sweet. There he made for them a statute and an ordinance, and there he proved them; and he said, If thou wilt diligently hearken to the voice of Jehovah thy God, and wilt do that which is right in his eyes, and wilt give ear to his commandments, and keep all his statutes, I will put none of the diseases upon thee, which I have put upon the Egyptians: for I am Jehovah that healeth thee. And they came to Elim, where

were twelve springs of water, and threescore and ten palm-trees: and they encamped there by the waters."

Exodus 15:22-27 ASV

Have you ever seen a movie, cartoon, or television show showing someone stranded in the desert? They are typically weak, thin, and crawling on the ground out of sheer exhaustion and the inability to bear their weight on their legs. They have dry wrinkly skin, parched cracked lips, and often have trouble speaking due to the dehydration. When they get to a water source, they appear so relieved and they drink it up as quickly as possible. Maybe you haven't seen a show like that, but I'm sure you've exercised hard, sweating out your body's water, getting dry cotton mouth, and feeling your heart pounding. Or you've gone many hours without something to drink and feel parched, and fatigued, with a headache and body ache. These are all classic signs of dehydration, and as you have felt, are uncomfortable.

We lose water through breathing, sweating, and digestion, so it is very important to rehydrate and replenish the body by eating foods that contain it, and drinking water multiple times per day. When you are dehydrated, you can feel sluggish, tired, bloated, and your skin can appear dry and wrinkly. Dehydration can also cause palpitations and make your heart race. It can cause very elevated blood pressures followed by dropped or low blood pressures if you go without water too long.

Water is essential for life. Our bodies are 70 percent water; the brain itself is 85 percent water, the blood is 80 percent water, and muscle is 70 percent water. The body uses water to regulate temperature, maintain bodily functions, and balance the cells and tissue. Water helps to flush our kidneys, keep the skin tight and looking good, is necessary for blood flow which helps the heart and blood pressure, and is necessary for digestion to prevent constipation. Most of the medical issues my patients come to see me about are connected to dehydration or not getting an adequate amount of water in each day. This is also why you often get a 2-pound bag of saline or fluid when you are in the hospital or Emergency Room; doctors know that having more fluid in the body can help with relaxation of the heart and blood vessels and aid in the healing process.

Although water is great for quenching your thirst, it has many other medical benefits. It helps to keep your tissues moist and lubricated. It can help in the joints, acting as a cushion or lubricant, and helping to protect the spinal cord. It helps to flush the body and remove waste and toxins through sweating, urinating, and bowel movements. It also helps to digest and break down food to release minerals and nutrients, essential for cell regeneration and muscle use. I can tell my patients aren't drinking enough water when they have slight swelling in their ankles. When the body is dehydrated, it will retain water as much as possible. This retained water often is stored in the ankles. I tell my patients who complain of non-pitting swollen ankles to drink more water so that their body doesn't have to retain it.

My patients often ask me, "How much water do I need each day?" Previously, experts suggested 8 glasses of water as the recommended daily intake, but how many ounces was that glass and what was the time frame for drinking those glasses? It turns out that 8 glasses of water per day is actually not an accurate calculation of how much water to drink, as some people need more water than others. Basically, the required amount is based on mass (weight and size); the larger you are, the more water you need. To calculate how much water your body needs, take your weight and divide it by 2. That number represents how many ounces of water you should drink daily, at a minimum. For example, if a person weighs 160 pounds, the calculation of water intake would be 160/2 = 80. So, they should drink at least 80 ounces of water each day. I know that sounds like a lot, but it is what is needed to replenish the amount of water that is lost each day. To convert that to bottles of water, take that number (in our example it is 80) and divide that by 16: 80/16 = 5 bottles minimum each day. This can be easier to accomplish when you break it down throughout the day: 1 bottle for breakfast, 1 bottle during the midmorning, 1 bottle for lunch, 1 bottle for afternoon snack, and 1 bottle for dinner. Another way to make this easier is to carry a large jug of water and put hash marks on the bottle corresponding to different times throughout the day. You will know when you are drinking enough water when you notice your urine is clear or yellowish clear (dark bright yellow or strong smelling urine is a sign of dehydration), your stools come out easily without straining, your mouth and eyes don't feel dry or itchy, and your skin is well hydrated and not dry or itchy. If you have any of the above-listed symptoms, you are likely not drinking enough water.

If you don't like water, get bored with drinking it, or feel like you are lacking taste, you can infuse your water with fruits like oranges, lemons, limes, or berries and herbs like mint or rosemary. Since water has no calories, it does not cause weight gain unlike sugary drinks like soda or fruit juice. You can drink as much plain or infused water as you'd like without worrying about it affecting your waistline!

Meditate Day and Night

"But whoever drinks of the water that I will give him will never be thirsty gain. The water that I will give him will become in him a spring of water welling up to eternal life.

John 4:14 NIV

"They shall not hunger or thirst, neither scorching wind nor sun shall strike them, for he who has pity on them will lead them, and by springs of water will guide them."

Isaiah 49:10 ESV

"Jesus stood up and cried out,
'If anyone thirsts, let him come to me and drink.
Whoever believes in me, as the scripture has said,
out of his heart will flow rivers of living water.'"

John 7:37-38 ESV

Practice What You Preach

List your weight, then divide it by 2. Divide this number by 16 to figure out how many bottles of water you need daily.

_____ lbs. / 2 = _____ ounces of water

_____ ounces of water / 16 = _____ bottles of water daily

List your favorite fruit and herb combinations to infuse your water.

_____

_____

_____

Challenge yourself to drink only water for 10 days (no sodas, juice, alcohol, or other beverages), and write down the differences you notice in weight, energy, skin, digestion, bathroom habits (urinary frequency or bowel habit changes), hair growth and strength, joint improvement, etc.

_____

_____

6

Spend More Quality Time with Family

"Don't be harsh or impatient with an older man. Talk to him as you would your own father, and to the younger men as your brothers. Reverently honor an older woman as you would your mother, and the younger women as sisters. Take care of widows who are destitute. If a widow has family members to take care of her, let them learn that religion begins at their own doorstep and that they should pay back with gratitude some of what they have received. This pleases God immensely. You can tell a legitimate widow by the way she has put all her hope in God, praying to him constantly for the needs of others as well as her own. But a widow who exploits people's emotions and pocketbooks—well, there's nothing to her.

Tell these things to the people so that they will do the right thing in their extended family. Anyone who neglects to care for family members in need repudiates the faith. That's worse than refusing to believe in the first place."

1 Timothy 5:1-8 MSG

I think back to times in my life where I celebrated large milestones like graduations, winning competitions, and having children. I also can recall some of the hardest times in my life like losing my grandfather, receiving a devastating diagnosis, or getting results of a failed test or a school rejection letter. The underlying thread in all of these situations was my family members cheering me on in victory, and comforting me in times of grief. I have come to learn, in my short time here on earth, that interpersonal connections with others, typically family and close friends, are essential for emotional and even physical well-being.

Humans have a basic need to feel love and acceptance from family and peers. Relationships are important to developing a sense of self, and emotions and behaviors are shaped by prior interactions and relationships with others. Love and relationships can affect physical and mental well-being. People can feel depressed and anxious and suffer from insomnia when relationships sour. There have also been documented cases where someone was in a coma, and when their loved one came closer, suddenly the comatose person started to improve in their vitals and brain activity. Because relationships are so crucial to the well-being of humans, it is a very important secret to divine health. Families are the first set of relationships we are introduced to at birth, and the impact of family weighs heavily on all aspects of our lives.

Family members are the people who know you the most. This can be a family of origin, a family of marriage, or a family that is not blood-related at all. In most cases, family has been around you most, if not all, of your life and have been present for all of the milestones that have occurred, both positive and negative. There is no bond like that of family. A mother's love is unparalleled and a father's love is unmatched. Though siblings often have a rivalry, they can be your biggest supporters and rally behind you at times when no one is there. I always find it amazing to watch siblings fight with each other, but stick up for each other when someone outside of the family unit confronts them. Don't discount other family members like cousins, godparents, and close family friends. Technically, any individuals that have supported or assisted you in your life can be considered family, blood relatives or not. Families are often our biggest supporters and help us financially, emotionally, and physically.

It is imperative that we give time to the ones who love us the most. Do not forget the power of family; they can make life easier at times, and their support is necessary and proven to be beneficial. Studies show that time with a mother can lower stress levels and that children and adolescents who spend more time with siblings and family get better grades, have fewer behavioral issues, and are less likely to participate in crime and violent activities. Family is important because they provide support and security; they love and understand you unconditionally. They help you make decisions whether that be through advice or example, even if that example is what not to do, as the best experience is sometimes learned secondhand. Family helps to mold and make us into our future selves.

People may forget what you gave them, but they will never forget time spent together. The more time you spend with people, the better chance you have of making memorable experiences. Sometimes quality time is more important than quantity of time, but studies have shown that quantity fosters the quality. We know that families with young children often spend more time together because young children need guidance and care, but it is important to continue to spend time with family as children become teenagers, and even into their adulthood. Family members need more face to face time, and less screen time and Facebook!

Though we work hard to be able to afford things, it is time spent that is often more memorable. We spend 40 hours or more at work, 60 hours sleeping, and 15 hours completing household tasks each week. That doesn't leave a lot of time for family, but by setting aside time each week, you can ensure you spend quality time with your family. Try sitting down together for a meal without cell phones for at least 30 minutes a day. Schedule a game night. Try exercising together. Start a book club in the family. Ask open-ended questions to foster conversation. Listen more than speaking. Be sure to include your family in the planning of the activities you will incorporate during quality time. Try to do something that each family member enjoys, even if you don't like the activity. If the kids love to play video games, try to set aside time to learn how to play, and the whole family can play together. If your wife likes the theater or going to shows, find a show that the family can go to together.

Try to spend time with the entire family, but also try to spend time with each individual so that they feel like they get their own special time. I will never forget the joy I felt each Tuesday as a pre-teen, when my dad would take me out to my piano lessons and after, we would go out to lunch or to the movies, or the record store. I looked forward to those times and I learned so much about my dad, his family of origin and upbringing. It was during those times that he taught me how to be an upstanding citizen, giving advice about experiences that have shaped my life. He taught me that a man should walk on the outside of the sidewalk to protect the lady from cars or splashed water and that a man should always sit facing the door in a restaurant so that they can watch your back. I cherished those times with my dad, and thank him each chance I get, as those valuable lessons and the time he spent with me, molded me into who I am today. Experiences like these benefited me emotionally by making me feel valued and teaching me what to expect from a man. I have chosen an excellent husband who spoils me and teaches my daughter the same concepts, so hopefully she will be able to choose a good mate and keep the pattern going.

Fathers, spend time with your sons. Show them how to be a man, how to work hard, and how to treat women. Mothers, spend time with your daughters. Teach them how to be ladies and carry themselves in a manner that is upstanding. I will never forget the time my mother spent with me teaching me how to cook, how to work hard, how to pay attention to details, how to help others, how to be a great wife and homemaker while working full-time, and how to love unconditionally. I remember my mom taking me and my siblings to amusement parks, and riding rides with us, laughing and having a good time. She took us to the movies and to ballets, helping us to develop a love of the arts, and taught us manners and how to present ourselves in public. These experiences are the things I remember, not the gifts or presents she bought me. Families need your presence more than they need your presents.

Spouses should also look to spend time with each other without the kids. The things you did to attract your spouse have to be continued to maintain and foster that relationship, so it can continue to flourish. Sometimes you have to actually schedule date night or family time, and refuse to let anything get in the way of that precious and valuable time. These moments are essential to healthy relationships and can't be made up. One of the most profound things my parents taught me was to live life without regrets, and I can tell you without question that you will not regret the time you spend with your family.

Hug and show affection to your family every day. Each time you leave the house or your family's presence, tell them you love them and show affection. Positive physical touch and affection help to lower stress hormones and release endorphins in the brain that make you feel good mentally and physically; we all know how warm and fuzzy we feel after giving and receiving a good hug or embrace. Never let the sun go down on your anger; work through disagreements and misunderstandings as soon as possible, as life is too short. We only get one family. I am reminded of a story Patti LaBelle told about her sister who was dying of cancer and asked Patti to make her a sandwich. Patti had just come off the road and told her sister she was tired and would make it for her the next day. The following day she made the sandwich, and when she called to tell her she was bringing it by, she found out her sister had just passed away. Patti talks about how that weighed so heavily on her. She performed the song "If You Asked Me To," in memory of her sister and the music video was made after the funeral. Now she encourages others, as I am doing here, to make the most of each moment you have with your loved ones here on earth. We know that time is fleeting, we only have one life to live with limited moments, so we should make the most of our time here on earth. James 4:14 (NASB) says, "*You do not know what your life will be like tomorrow, you are just a vapor that appears for a little while and then vanishes away.*" You never know the last time you will interact with, see, hug, or tell them that you love them, so make an effort to do it today and every day.

Meditate Day and Night

"Children are a heritage from the Lord, offspring a reward from Him. Like arrows in the hands of a warrior are children born in one's youth. Blessed is the man whose quiver is full of them. They will not be put to shame when they contend with their opponents in court."

Psalm 127:3-5 NIV

"A wise son brings joy to his father, but a foolish man despises his mother."

Proverbs 15:20 NIV

"Your offspring shall be like the dust of the earth, and you shall spread abroad to the west and to the east and to the north and to the south, and in you and your offspring shall all the families of the earth be blessed."

Genesis 28:14 ESV

Practice What You Preach

List three things you can do with your family this week.

List three great and unique attributes of your spouse, children, and/or family, and how you will let them know you appreciate them this week.

Plan a vacation or staycation with your family that everyone will enjoy. Write the details and contact information here for reference.

Use this page as a scrap book to post pictures and souvenirs of your family vacation/staycation.

7

Tend to Your Mental Health

*"When the cares of my heart are many,
your consolations cheer my soul."*

Psalm 94:19 ESV

We cannot address whole-man health without addressing mental health issues. Although there is a large continuum of mental health disorders, from disorders like dysthymia (chronic persistent depressive disorder), to disorders like schizophrenia with delusions and hallucinations, the most commonly seen mental health disorders are depression and anxiety. There are more than three million cases of depression and anxiety each year. These two disorders are often diagnosed together in patients, and if not recognized and treated early, can lead to more health problems, both physical and mental. Problems with depression and anxiety can often manifest through difficulty sleeping, both sleeping too much, and the inability to sleep well at all.

We are one body with three parts: the physical, spiritual, and mental. When one part of the body is ill, it affects the other parts as well. It is not uncommon to see someone who is dealing with a chronic illness also deal with depression. Living with chronic disease can be disheartening, difficult, and life-altering. Often, when people realize that they have to be on medications chronically, or that they will have limitations to their lifestyle, they become depressed, which can cause additional medical complications. For example, people who are overly stressed and depressed can have tension in their neck, shoulders, and upper back leading to spasms, pain, arthritis, and limited range of motion. The pain, which is sometimes difficult to treat, along with the limited motion, changes a patient's lifestyle causing an even deeper depressive state. This becomes a vicious cycle that can be difficult to treat.

Often, doctors put patients on antidepressants while treating certain conditions that cause pain, as the medications help lower the pain threshold, and also help treat the depression and insomnia that can be concurrent. Most antidepressants also serve as anxiolytics (anti-anxiety medications) and also as sleeping medication to treat insomnia. The most common antidepressants/anxiolytics are SSRI's (selective serotonin reuptake Inhibitors) like Paxil, Prozac, Zoloft, Celexa, and

Lexapro), and there are other types that are all used to treat the problems listed above.

In today's society, mental illness has a negative stigma, while physical illness does not always carry that stigma. Anxiety, depression, and some of the other mental illnesses are often the result of a chemical imbalance of the neurotransmitters in the brain. The aim of medication is to reset this chemical imbalance. It is important to remember that the imbalance present with depression is similar to having an imbalance in the pancreas which leads to diabetes. Since we do not shun illnesses like diabetes, we should refrain from negative thinking regarding mental illness, especially within ourselves.

The first step to treating any illness, including mental illness, is acknowledging that there is a problem. If you are having trouble sleeping, have a short temper, crying spells, are feeling down or in despair, or feeling overly anxious, seek counsel from a doctor and therapist/counselor while improving your diet and increasing exercise. There are multiple tests that can be taken to screen for anxiety and depression. Some are listed in the "Practice what You Preach" section.

After you recognize that you are dealing with a mental illness, your doctor can either monitor you or put you on medication. However, it is important to address mental health issues with a variety of treatments. Even if you are started on medication, you can best treat the mental illness with therapy (either group or individual), healthy diet, exercise, and getting enough sleep. Multiple treatments are available because there are multiple causes of mental illness and situations that can worsen those symptoms. By having a variety of treatment options, all of the causes can be addressed: physical, mental, emotional, and interpersonal. Social interaction like going out with friends or attending events is also paramount in the treatment of anxiety or depression.

If you are started on medication for management, the medicine has to be monitored. If the medicine is not working, either because it is too strong, not strong enough, or not effective, the doses must be changed carefully by a trained, licensed physician. I encourage all of my patients taking any medications, but especially mental disorder medications, to never stop taking your medication abruptly without direction of your doctor. Many of these medications have to be weaned down to limit side effects, withdrawal, and other medical problems. Many patients stop taking their medicine because they are feeling better and end up back in the doctor's office with other recurrent problems because the medication was working to balance the hormones and neurotransmitters, which made them feel better until they stopped the medicine and the chemicals became unbalanced again. This is not to discourage you or to imply that once on medication you have to stay on medication. Most doctors keep patients on antidepressants for 3-6 months, then re-evaluate to see if the mediation can be weaned and stopped, or if it needs to continue.

It is important to see your doctor regularly while taking these medications, as sometimes there are labs and other testing such as thyroid testing, testing of blood sugar, or blood pressure levels that must be performed while taking the medication. It is also important to tell your doctor about any therapy or counseling sessions you attend. This is considered an integral part of your treatment plan and your therapist and doctor should be aware of the treatment plan from each.

The following "Practice What You Preach" section includes depression and anxiety screening tools that doctors use to help quantify and determine the severity of depression and anxiety.

Practice What You Preach

K10 Test

These questions concern how you have been feeling over the past 30 days. Tick a box below each question that best represents how you have been.

1. During the last 30 days, about how often did you feel tired out for no good reason?				
1. None of the time	2. A little of the time	3. Some of the time	4. Most of the time	5. All of the time

2. During the last 30 days, about how often did you feel nervous?				
1. None of the time	2. A little of the time	3. Some of the time	4. Most of the time	5. All of the time

3. During the last 30 days, about how often did you feel so nervous that nothing could calm you down?				
1. None of the time	2. A little of the time	3. Some of the time	4. Most of the time	5. All of the time

4. During the last 30 days, about how often did you feel hopeless?				
1. None of the time	2. A little of the time	3. Some of the time	4. Most of the time	5. All of the time

5. During the last 30 days, about how often did you feel restless or fidgety?				
1. None of the time	2. A little of the time	3. Some of the time	4. Most of the time	5. All of the time

6. During the last 30 days, about how often did you feel so restless you could not sit still?				
1. None of the time	2. A little of the time	3. Some of the time	4. Most of the time	5. All of the time

7. During the last 30 days, about how often did you feel depressed?				
1. None of the time	2. A little of the time	3. Some of the time	4. Most of the time	5. All of the time

8. During the last 30 days, about how often did you feel that everything was an effort?				
1. None of the time	2. A little of the time	3. Some of the time	4. Most of the time	5. All of the time

9. During the last 30 days, about how often did you feel so sad that nothing could cheer you up?				
1. None of the time	2. A little of the time	3. Some of the time	4. Most of the time	5. All of the time

10. During the last 30 days, about how often did you feel worthless?				
1. None of the time	2. A little of the time	3. Some of the time	4. Most of the time	5. All of the time

Kessler Psychological Distress Scale (K10)
Source: Kessler R. Professor of Health Care Policy, Harvard Medical School, Boston, USA.

This is a 10-item questionnaire intended to yield a global measure of distress based on questions about anxiety and depressive symptoms that a person has experienced in the most recent 4 week period.

Why use the K10
The use of a consumer self-report measure is a desirable method of assessment because it is a genuine attempt on the part of the clinician to collect information on the patient's current condition and to establish a productive dialogue. When completing the K10 the consumer should be provided with privacy.
(Information sourced from the NSW Mental health Outcomes and Assessment Training (MH-OAT) facilitator's Manual, NSW Health Department 2001)

How to administer the questionnaire
As a general rule, patients who rate most commonly "Some of the time" or "All of the time" categories are in need of a more detailed assessment. Referral information should be provided to these individuals. Patients who rate most commonly "A little of the time" or "None of the time" may also benefit from early intervention and promotional information to assist raising awareness of the conditions of depression and anxiety as well as strategies to prevent future mental health issues.

(Information sourced from the NSW Mental health Outcomes and Assessment Training (MH-OAT) facilitator's Manual, NSW Health Department 2001)

If you scored more than 20 points, this may represent manifestations of depression and/or anxiety, and you should make an appointment as soon as possible with your primary care physician and/or a licensed therapist. Please bring a copy of this test for your healthcare provider to go over, and formulate a treatment plan.

Beck's Depression Inventory

This depression inventory can be self-scored. The scoring scale is at the end of the questionnaire.

1.
   - 0 I do not feel sad.
   - 1 I feel sad
   - 2 I am sad all the time and I can't snap out of it.
   - 3 I am so sad and unhappy that I can't stand it.

2.
   - 0 I am not particularly discouraged about the future.
   - 1 I feel discouraged about the future.
   - 2 I feel I have nothing to look forward to.
   - 3 I feel the future is hopeless and that things cannot improve.

3.
   - 0 I do not feel like a failure.
   - 1 I feel I have failed more than the average person.
   - 2 As I look back on my life, all I can see is a lot of failures.
   - 3 I feel I am a complete failure as a person.

4.
   - 0 I get as much satisfaction out of things as I used to.
   - 1 I don't enjoy things the way I used to.
   - 2 I don't get real satisfaction out of anything anymore.
   - 3 I am dissatisfied or bored with everything.

5.
   - 0 I don't feel particularly guilty
   - 1 I feel guilty a good part of the time.
   - 2 I feel quite guilty most of the time.
   - 3 I feel guilty all of the time.

6.
   - 0 I don't feel I am being punished.
   - 1 I feel I may be punished.
   - 2 I expect to be punished.
   - 3 I feel I am being punished.

7.
   - 0 I don't feel disappointed in myself.
   - 1 I am disappointed in myself.
   - 2 I am disgusted with myself.
   - 3 I hate myself.

8.
   - 0 I don't feel I am any worse than anybody else.
   - 1 I am critical of myself for my weaknesses or mistakes.
   - 2 I blame myself all the time for my faults.
   - 3 I blame myself for everything bad that happens.

9.
   - 0 I don't have any thoughts of killing myself.
   - 1 I have thoughts of killing myself, but I would not carry them out.
   - 2 I would like to kill myself.
   - 3 I would kill myself if I had the chance.

10.
   - 0 I don't cry any more than usual.
   - 1 I cry more now than I used to.
   - 2 I cry all the time now.
   - 3 I used to be able to cry, but now I can't cry even though I want to.

11.
- 0   I am no more irritated by things than I ever was.
- 1   I am slightly more irritated now than usual.
- 2   I am quite annoyed or irritated a good deal of the time.
- 3   I feel irritated all the time.

12.
- 0   I have not lost interest in other people.
- 1   I am less interested in other people than I used to be.
- 2   I have lost most of my interest in other people.
- 3   I have lost all of my interest in other people.

13.
- 0   I make decisions about as well as I ever could.
- 1   I put off making decisions more than I used to.
- 2   I have greater difficulty in making decisions more than I used to.
- 3   I can't make decisions at all anymore.

14.
- 0   I don't feel that I look any worse than I used to.
- 1   I am worried that I am looking old or unattractive.
- 2   I feel there are permanent changes in my appearance that make me look unattractive
- 3   I believe that I look ugly.

15.
- 0   I can work about as well as before.
- 1   It takes an extra effort to get started at doing something.
- 2   I have to push myself very hard to do anything.
- 3   I can't do any work at all.

16.
- 0   I can sleep as well as usual.
- 1   I don't sleep as well as I used to.
- 2   I wake up 1-2 hours earlier than usual and find it hard to get back to sleep.
- 3   I wake up several hours earlier than I used to and cannot get back to sleep.

17.
- 0   I don't get more tired than usual.
- 1   I get tired more easily than I used to.
- 2   I get tired from doing almost anything.
- 3   I am too tired to do anything.

18.
- 0   My appetite is no worse than usual.
- 1   My appetite is not as good as it used to be.
- 2   My appetite is much worse now.
- 3   I have no appetite at all anymore.

19.
- 0   I haven't lost much weight, if any, lately.
- 1   I have lost more than five pounds.
- 2   I have lost more than ten pounds.
- 3   I have lost more than fifteen pounds.

20.
- 0   I am no more worried about my health than usual.
- 1   I am worried about physical problems like aches, pains, upset stomach, or constipation.
- 2   I am very worried about physical problems and it's hard to think of much else.
- 3   I am so worried about my physical problems that I cannot think of anything else.

21.
- 0   I have not noticed any recent change in my interest in sex.
- 1   I am less interested in sex than I used to be.
- 2   I have almost no interest in sex.
- 3   I have lost interest in sex completely.

INTERPRETING THE BECK DEPRESSION INVENTORY

Now that you have completed the questionnaire, add up the score for each of the twenty-one questions by counting the number to the right of each question you marked. The highest possible total for the whole test would be sixty-three. This would mean you circled number three on all twenty-one questions. Since the lowest possible score for each question is zero, the lowest possible score for the test would be zero. This would mean you circles zero on each question. You can evaluate your depression according to the Table below.

Total Score	Levels of Depression
1-10	These ups and downs are considered normal
11-16	Mild mood disturbance
17-20	Borderline clinical depression
21-30	Moderate depression
31-40	Severe depression
over 40	Extreme depression

This is another depression and anxiety screening tool. If you scored more than 16 points, please contact a healthcare provider so that they can formulate a treatment plan for you.

Don't be discouraged if you are dealing with anxiety, depression, or any other mental illnesses. Mental illness is very common, affecting 1 in 5 Americans each year. Symptoms can be as mild as the blues with Seasonal Affect Disorder, or severe with audio and visual hallucinations, which impair the activities of daily living. Treatment plans are best when they are personalized for each individual, and work better when are treated early.

Meditate Day and Night

"God is our refuge and strength, an ever-present help in trouble. Therefore we will not fear, though the earth give way and the mountains fall into the heart of the sea, though its waters roar and foam and the mountains quake with their surging. There is a river whose streams make glad the city of God, the holy place where the Most High dwells. God is within her, she will not fall; God will help her at break of day."

Psalm 46:1-5 NIV

"Do not be anxious about anything, but in every situation by prayer and petition with thanksgiving present your requests to God. And the peace of God, which transcends all understanding, will guard your hearts and your minds in Christ Jesus."

Philippians 4:6-7 NIV

"Do not be conformed to this world, but be transformed by the renewal of your mind, that by testing you may discern what is the will of God, what is good sand acceptable and perfect."

Romans 12:2 NKJV

8

Take Your Vitamins and Medicines as Prescribed

"By the river on its bank, on one side and on the other, will grow all kinds of trees for food. Their leaves will not wither and their fruit will not fail. They will bear every month because their water flows from the sanctuary, and their fruit will be for food and their leaves for healing."

Ezekiel 47:12 NASB

With the modernization of western culture and technology came improvements in treatment of medical conditions and medications. There are a variety of medications to treat various medical conditions. For example, there are nine different categories/classes of medication to treat hypertension (high blood pressure), with multiple medications in each category. Your doctor has been trained to know how each medication works in the body and how it can benefit your medical condition. Your doctor chooses medications based on how they work in the body, your other medical conditions, possible side effects, and even how easy it would be to take the medication. For example, some medications must be taken 5 times a day, whereas other medications can be taken twice a day. Consequently, your doctor may prescribe the twice-a-day medication because it is easier for the patient to remember a pill twice a day over five times a day. Your doctor will also take pricing into account when prescribing a medication. There are some formulations of medicine that have an extended release version. Those medications should be taken once a day, so it is easier for patients to remain compliant with taking the medication. However, it is important to remember that these once-a-day extended release tablets are often more expensive than a multiple time a day medications. Things like cost, effectiveness, and ease of taking the medication should be discussed with your doctor.

Vitamins have also become very popular and can be purchased without a prescription. Vitamins are supplements taken to build up the tissues, cells, and organs in the body. It is recommended to take a daily vitamin to replenish the electrolytes, nutrients, and minerals that are lost through our normal body function. Because western society is not as focused on a plant based diet, many of us are lacking in nutrients and depend on vitamins to replenish these minerals. Schedule an appointment to discuss medications and vitamins with your doctor before adding or changing them. Certain vitamins can affect medical conditions and may negatively interact with prescribed medications.

Doctors recommend, and many times prefer, treating certain disease processes with lifestyle modifications like diet, weight loss, and stress management. When these modifications do not work or are not effective, prescription medication may be necessary.

Medications should not be stopped or adjusted without instruction from your doctor, as some medications require tapering for safety. Do not take advice or adjust your medication based on another person's dosing. I once had a patient tell me that his blood pressure medication dosage was too strong because he was on 160mg but his friend was only on 10mg, so he stopped taking it. What he didn't realize was that the 10mg his friend was taking was the highest dosage of the medication in that class, but the 160mg I prescribed was actually the lowest dosage in the class of medication I prescribed. Stopping medication or adjusting medication on your own can result in worsening disease, progression to other conditions, or adverse reactions like withdrawal. If you do want to discontinue a medication or adjust it, please make an appointment to speak with your doctor as soon as possible. You may be able to discuss a plan to see if you are able to wean down on the medication or change it to something else.

I always recommend that patients keep a list of medications they have been on in the past, what medications they are currently prescribed, what medications have been changed, how any changes should be implemented, and if the medication is still necessary or if it can be weaned or stopped. Before you leave your doctor's office, be sure to have a full understanding of times you should be taking your medicine, if it needs to be taken with food or on an empty stomach, other supplements or medications it should not be mixed with, possible side effects, and what to expect from taking the medication. For example, should you expect your blood pressure to go down, but possibly your heart rate to go up while taking a medication?

When patients are seen by multiple doctors and specialists, one doctor may not know what medications another doctor has prescribed. You don't want to have any negative interactions with medications, so please be sure all of your doctors know what medications other doctors prescribe or have changed. By keeping the updated list available, all of the doctors on your healthcare team can know what is going on with your health in order to work together to help you have the best health possible.

The discussion of multiple doctors and specialists broaches another medical issue that is too commonly seen: polypharmacy. Polypharmacy is when a person is taking too much medication, some of which may be interacting with other medications or causing other problems. For example, I had a patient once who was taking a blood pressure medication, and one of the side effects of that medication was constriction in the lungs. It is a great blood pressure medication, but it is possible that whoever prescribed the medicine didn't know the patient also had asthma. Once he began taking that medication, which did help the blood pressure, he started having more shortness of breath and asthma attacks. He then went to see his pulmonologist (lung doctor) who put him on two other medications to control the asthma. One of the asthma medications had a side effect of dyspepsia (indigestion and acid reflux), so another doctor put him on an acid reducer medication. When he came to me, I looked at his medication profile, went through his history and determined that all of these new symptoms and medications were coming from the blood pressure medication. After changing his blood pressure medication, his asthma improved and he was able to come off the extra asthma medications. This improved the acid reflux, and he was able to come off the acid reflux medications. His blood pressure is now well controlled with one pill and lifestyle changes. He has no problems with acid reflux or asthma attacks. Polypharmacy is frequent among elderly patients who have multiple specialists and multiple health conditions requiring treatment. I don't say this to imply that people should not take medications, or to cause fear, but I want you to be aware that all medication, even over-the-counter pills and supplements, have side effects. Your health care team needs to know about all of your conditions and medications to come up with the best treatment plan for you.

It is important to know the current names, dosages, and frequency of the medication you are taking, and have up to date pharmacy information available if needed. Many of the medications available are made by different manufacturers and can appear to be different, so telling your doctor, "I take the little triangle shaped purple pill," does not help us in identifying the medication. It is also best to bring your medications with you to your doctor's appointments so that your doctor can go over the medication if needed.

If you notice a change in your medication that you were not aware of, please contact your doctor's office immediately as it could be a transcription error (the medication was written or read incorrectly), a pharmacy filling error, or the manufacturer may have changed, resulting in a different looking pill. You can take the pill to your doctor or pharmacist for confirmation that it is the correct pill.

When you need a refill on your medication, do not wait until the day you run out to fill it or request a refill, as most doctor's offices require 24-72 hours to be able to fill the medication. Always check with your pharmacy first to make sure there are not refills on hold, which will bypass the additional step of calling the doctor's office. It is best to call for refills the week prior to running out of the medication to ensure the doctor has time to send the prescription, and the pharmacy has time to fill the prescription before you run out of the medication.

Your pharmacist is also an important factor in your medical care and can answer questions about the medications, what interactions they may have with other foods or supplements, and how to best follow your doctor's instructions in taking the medication. Your pharmacist should be able to give you a complete list of medications, past and currently prescribed. It is a good idea to keep a list of those medications handy, especially when going to a doctor's appointment so that the doctor can see the list and check to make sure it matches their current list.

Meditate Day and Night

"No longer drink only water, but use a little wine for the sake of your stomach and your frequent ailments."

1 Timothy 5:23 ESV

"Through the middle of the street of the city; also on either side of the river, the tree of life with its twelve kinds of fruit, yielding its fruit each month. The leaves of the tree were for the healing of the nation."

Revelation 22:2 ESV

"Now Isaiah had said, 'Let them take a cake of figs and apply it to the boil, that he may recover.'"

Isaiah 38:21 NASB

Medication List

Name	Dosage Frequency	Condition	Treating Physician

Supplement List

Name	Dosage Frequency	Condition	Treating Physician

Practice What You Preach

1. Schedule a doctor's appointment to go over your list of medications. Find out what each medication is for and at what frequency they should be taken to optimize their effectiveness. Also, ask about food or drink interactions that may interfere with the medication to ensure that those interactions do not worsen any of your other medical conditions.

2. Ask your doctor if any medications can be weaned and stopped and if not, how long they suspect you will be taking the medication.

3. Consider holistic approaches like taking supplements and using food as adjuncts to your medication regimen. This may optimize your health benefits and limit the amount of medication you have to take if approved and monitored by your doctor.

9

Relax, Smile, and Be Merry

*"A cheerful heart is good medicine,
but a crushed spirit dries up the bones."*

Proverbs 17:22 NIV

The need for relaxation has never been more apparent than now. We live in a time when violence is paramount, and poverty impacts even first world countries. Unfortunately, many people are overcome by a lack of basic provisions. People are working harder to make ends meet, and are often doing the work of multiple people. This leads to burnout, depression, anxiety, trouble sleeping, weight gain, and physical illness.

Relaxation is more than going on vacation, enjoying a hobby, or "vegging out." Relaxation is defined as the state of being free from tension and anxiety. It is a process that decreases the effects of stress on your mind and body. Relaxation helps you to cope with the stressors of everyday life. As discussed in the previous chapter on meditation, studies have shown that medical conditions like heart disease, chronic pain, and metabolic regulation can be positively impacted by relaxation techniques.

Relaxation techniques include but are not limited to deep breathing, meditation, rhythmic exercise, yoga, exercise, sleeping/napping, quiet introspection, stretching, aromatherapy, drinking herbal teas, massage, acupressure/acupuncture, listening to music, reading a book, spending time with family and friends, and anything that takes your mind away from the stressors of the day. Relaxation techniques vary based on individuals and can even vary at different times. Today I may relax by taking an invigorating run, and tomorrow I may relax by taking a nice bubble bath. Some people find loud music relaxing while others seek out silence and solitude.

However it's done, relaxation helps to ease tight sore muscles, helps to slow down the heart rate and lower blood pressure. Stress causes the release of stress hormones in the body that can increase weight gain, lower immune function, clog the arteries, slow the lymphatic system, increase blood pressure and blood sugar, and cause or worsen neurological disorders. It is not uncommon for people to have headaches when they become stressed, which results in more tension in the neck, upper shoulders, and back. When stress levels are high, it can cause a flare of shingles or multiple sclerosis in people with those disease processes, and the flares can be debilitating. Stress is unfortunately such a big portion of our lives, that I have devoted an entire chapter to it in this book to delve into more aspects of the effect of stress on the body, and how we can better handle it (see chapter 12).

Relaxation helps to boost our mood and can make us feel better. This leads to happiness and an increased satisfaction with life. Happiness is important because the quality of our lives is based on our emotions. Life is 10 percent what happens to us and 90 percent how we deal with what life brings. Happiness is contagious and by being happy, we can positively change others around us. Happiness is often manifested in a smile which can brighten a room, lighten burdens, and cause joy.

When we smile, the muscles in our faces contract and cause a positive feedback loop to the brain that reinforces the joyous feeling. A scientist stated that smiling stimulates the brain's reward mechanism more than chocolate. When we feel good, we smile, and when we smile it tells our brain, which feels good and causes a repetitive cycle.

Meditate Day and Night

*"Then, because so many people were coming
and going that they did not even have a chance
to eat, he said to them 'come with me by yourselves
to a quiet place to get some rest."*

Mark 6:31 NIV

*"Remember the Sabbath day, to keep it holy. Six days you
shall labor, and do all your work, 10 but the seventh day
is a sabbath to the Lord your god. ON it you shall not do
any work, you or your son, or your daughter, your male
servant or your female servant or your livestock, or the
sojourner who is within your gates. For in six days the
Lord made heaven and earth, the sea, and all that is in
them, and rested on the seventh day. Therefore, the lord
blessed the sabbath day and made it holy."*

Exodus 20: 8-11 NASB

*"He makes me to lie down in green pastures,
He leads me beside quiet waters. He refreshes my soul."*

Psalm 23:2-3 NIV

"Come to me all you who've are weary and burdened, and I will give you rest. Take my yoke upon you and learn from me, for I am gentle and humble in heart and you will find rest for your souls. For my yoke is easy and my burden is light."

Matthew 11:28-30 NIV

"So it came about whenever the evil spirit from god came to Saul, David would take the harp and play it with his hand; and Saul would be refreshed and be well, and the evil spirit would depart from him."

1 Samuel 16:23 NASB

"How happy your people must be! How happy your officials, who continually stand before you and hear your wisdom."

2 Chronicles 9:7 NIV

Practice What You Preach

List some things that make you smile.

List at least 10 ways that you can relax:

List some ways you can see positivity in previous negative situations.

10
Get an Annual Physical

"I praise you, for I am fearfully and wonderfully made. Wonderful are your works; my soul knows it very well."

Psalm 139:14 ESV

Doctor's offices are filled with sick individuals seeking treatment for their ailments, but there are a growing number of people who come to the doctor when they are well. This number should be increasing as we in the medical profession now heavily promote the concept of annual wellness visits. Wellness visits are a form of secondary prevention that is defined as measures to end disease before it fully develops by reducing the number of new or severe cases of a disease. In this instance, the disease has already occurred in the community, and we use the history of the patient, location, age, gender, and family history to test for, and attempt to avoid development of, medical problems. Primary prevention is concerned with preventing the onset of disease by reducing how often and when the disease occurs. This involves interventions that are applied before there is any evidence of disease or injury and is most commonly done with vaccinations to prevent disease from occurring before it is even present. Tertiary prevention attempts to soften the impact and progression of an already ongoing illness or injury and is done by helping people manage long-term diseases and injuries to improve quality of life and life expectancy.

Examples of each type of prevention are listed here: Primary-immunizations to eradicate disease like polio, mumps, chicken pox, etc. and education about safe habits like eating well, exercising, and not smoking; Secondary-regular exams and screening tests to detect disease in its earliest stages, like mammograms to detect breast cancer, or PSAs to detect prostate cancer; Tertiary- rehabilitation programs and chronic disease management program like cardiac rehab after heart attack or heart failure, and diabetes education after diagnosis of disease. This also includes vocational rehab to retrain workers for new jobs after recovery from disease or illness, and support groups that allow members to share ideas and strategies to improve life while living with disease.

Secondary prevention wellness exams should be done annually whether you are sick or not. Actually, you should not wait until you are sick to see your doctor for your annual wellness exam, as the wellness exam and sick visit are billed differently. If you wait until you are sick to schedule the wellness exam, you may be charged more for both visits to occur. Wellness exams are crucial to overall improved health because prevention is the key to longevity. By having wellness exams, individuals can find potential problems before they occur, and if problems are found, they can be treated earlier which makes them easier to manage and hopefully eradicate. Most people don't know about wellness exams, or what to expect at them. By having knowledge of the exam, you can be more informed of what to look for and what questions to ask.

The wellness exam varies based on gender, age, geographical location, and past and family history. Although there are some differences, the similarities of a wellness exam include a thorough past medical, family, and social history, a physical exam, and preventative measures for the future. Next listed are some differences in physicals based on age and gender.

Newborn exams occur immediately after birth, at 1-2 weeks, and then 1-2 months. These consist of a full head to toe exam, paying close attention to the bones and joints, as these can uncover congenital (born with or genetic) processes like hip joint problems. Hearing exams are also conducted, as well as light reflex exams for the eyes. At these exams, primary prevention also occurs through immunizations.

Infant exams occur at 2 months, 4 months, 6 months, 9 months, 12 months, 15 months, 18 months, and 24 months. These exams consist of a full physical and checking for developmental milestones at each age. Anticipatory guidance also occurs to help ensure safety and prevent problems from occurring. Doctors provide reminders for seatbelt and car seat use, ask questions regarding smoke and fire detectors in the home, gun safety, toilet training, healthy diet, etc.

Childhood exams should occur yearly and include a full physical examination, immunizations, ongoing developmental milestone checks, and anticipatory guidance. Doctors discuss information such as limiting screen time, education on good and bad touches, bullying, educational issues like tutoring and studying tips, encouraging reading, dental visits, and exercise and physical activity.

Adolescent exams consist of the physical exam, immunizations, and education with anticipatory guidance. If the child is playing sports, which is encouraged if there are no issues that would cause problems with physical activity, a sports physical or clearance is completed. Education includes pubertal changes to the body, educational topics like studying and college prep, questions about friends and peer pressure, and avoidance of destructive behaviors like drugs, alcohol, violence, and sex education.

Exams for adults age 18-40 involve a physical exam, education, and when warranted, labs to screen for diseases like diabetes, kidney problems, and cholesterol. Education includes diet and exercise recommendations, smoking cessation if needed, and information regarding avoidance of high risk behaviors like excessive alcohol, drug use, and high risk sexual activity. For women over age 21, a Pap smear is conducted every 1-5 years based on presence of HPV (human papilloma virus). STD screening and testing can be done if warranted. Men in this age group do not have any required testing unless they are at high risk for diseases like diabetes or heart disease based on their history and family history.

Exams for adults age 40-65 involve a physical exam, labs when warranted, and screening. Men should be screened for prostate cancer with a digital rectal exam to feel the prostate, and possibly a PSA if warranted. Women should have their Pap smear every 3-5 years, and a mammogram every 1-2 years, along with a clinical breast exam. Women are also encouraged to do breast self-exams monthly to feel for any changes to the tissue in the breast or to the skin on the breast. Both men and women should have a screening colonoscopy at age 50 unless they are high risk for colon cancer or have a family history and in that case, it may be warranted earlier. This should be discussed with your doctor to determine the best time for your initial colonoscopy. Education should be given as well, to address issues like diet and exercise planning, smoking cessation if needed, avoidance of high risk activities, mental health screening to ensure there is no anxiety or depression that can affect lifestyle, and vision screening. Around this time, it is not uncommon for tertiary prevention to be done, as other medical issues are present and attempts are initiated or maintained to improve and prevent worsening of chronic disease.

Exams for adults over 65 include a full physical exam, mental health evaluation and screening, labs, and education. For women, Pap smears can be stopped over age 65, but mammograms and breast exams should continue to at least 75, or longer if there is family history or it is warranted. Men should continue their annual prostate exams, and may be referred to a urologist if there are any lower urinary tract symptoms like urinary frequency, increased urination at night, erectile dysfunction, or decreased sex drive. These can be symptoms of an enlarging prostate, which is common as men grow older. If the prostate enlarges and medication given by the primary care physician does not control it, they may be referred to a urologist for further testing and treatment. Skin exams should also occur, at least annually, for both men and women, to ensure there are no changing moles or skin lesions which could be malignant or precancerous. Mental exams consist of screening for depression and memory loss or dementia.

At 65, once a person enrolls in Medicare, a welcome to Medicare physical is done. This must occur before the patient turns 66, and is covered under the new Medicare plan. This exam is a safety and prevention check. A mini mental status exam is done to rule out memory loss and dementia. Safety checks are done to try to promote a healthy lifestyle, and avoid things like slipping and falling, which can increase the risk of hip fractures. They also make sure all screening exams have been completed: colonoscopy, mammogram, the last Pap smear if needed, EKG to rule out cardiac problems, and labs.

At all annual physicals, you should ask questions about how you can remain healthy over the upcoming year and get education about any chronic medical issues you may be facing. You should also go over any medication or supplements you are taking, and get recommendations on diet and exercise.

Annual physicals are extensive, but are necessary to prevent and screen for chronic disease. If disease is noted, all efforts are made to ensure correct management of the disease, and to improve or resolve it if possible. Do not wait until you are sick to see your doctor. For the sake of your health, schedule and attend your wellness exams. Prevention is the key to longevity and healthy lifestyle.

Meditate Day and Night

"He went to him and bound up his wounds, pouring on oil and wine. Then he set him on his own animal and brought him to an inn and took care of him.

Luke 10:34 ESV

"Is there no balm in Gilead? Is there no physician there? Why then has not the health of the daughter of my people been restored?"

Jeremiah 8:22 NAS

Practice What You Preach

1. Call your doctor and schedule your annual physical.

2. List any questions you need to discuss with your doctor about preventing medical conditions.

3. Write down any recommendations or education your doctor gives you to help improve your health.

4. Write down the dates of your screenings (labs, colonoscopy, mammogram, prostate check).

11

Treat Your Body as a Temple

"Or do you not know that your body is a temple of the Holy Spirit within you, whom you have from God? You are not your own, for you were bought with a price. So glorify God in your body."

1 Corinthians 6:19-20 ESV

A temple is defined as a building devoted to worship, or regarded as the dwelling place of a god or gods, or other objects of religious reverence. A physical temple is held to a higher level of esteem: people speak quietly around them, turn off their loud music, stop cursing in and around them, put out cigarettes in and around them, remove their hats as a sign of respect, and try to be on their best behavior. I'm sure you've heard someone say, "You can't do that in a church!" as they realize that the temple or church is a holy place.

We should treat our bodies the same way. Since our bodies are the temple of God, and the dwelling place not only for the spiritual deity, but also for our own trinity of mind, body, and spirit, we should treat our bodies with a high level of respect. We shouldn't do things to our body that will harm it or desecrate it. We shouldn't smoke, eat or drink in excess, and we should do our best to maintain the premises through healthy diet and exercise. Just as the physical temple is adorned with stained glass windows, pictures, and statues to beautify it, we should do our best to beautify our bodies as well.

We've all heard of churches raising money for the building fund to help maintain the physical appearance of the temple. In the same manner, we should set funds aside to maintain our appearance. It's ok to make a special fund for self-care. Things like getting your hair done, getting a manicure and pedicure, getting a massage, hiring a personal trainer, eating healthier organic foods, and getting skin treatments can all be categorized as self-care and are needed. Pampering yourself is often a want and not a need, as it will help you mentally and physically, but is not essential. Pampering can be done by getting new clothes that fit better, purchasing comfortable but stylish shoes, going on vacation, and buying self-help books. We know that when we look good, we feel good, and that helps us continue taking care of our temples. Have you noticed that after exercising consistently for a while, when someone compliments your weight loss or increased muscles and tone, you become more motivated to continue exercising, and sometimes even increase your exercise efforts to continue the changes in appearance?

What are some physical ways we can treat our body as a temple? By applying the 12 secrets revealed in this book: increasing water intake to hydrate the skin and organs to help them perform at a better level and look better, increasing exercise with the intent to not only look good, but to feel good. By decreasing stress and attending to our mental health, and by improving work/life balance and knowing how to detach and leave work at work. You honor your temple by maintaining your health and seeing your doctor regularly, and by being proactive and addressing tough issues early to keep them from building up and growing, making them harder to manage. By spending more time with family and loved ones. By challenging ourselves to do things we've never done before and things we never thought we could do. By keeping our brain active and continuing to learn something new every day. By practicing gratefulness and being thankful for what we have, don't have, and are working through and toward. By meditating daily and developing a deeper, more meaningful relationship with God. Finally, we can honor our temples by being mindful of our bodies, and not feeling guilty when we take care of it. Some people view self-care as selfish and proud, but it is actually selfless. Two famous sayings confirming the benefits of self-care are, "You can't fill from an empty cup," and "In the event of an emergency, put on your mask before attending to others." It is true that caring for yourself puts you in a better position to care for others.

Meditate Day and Night

"I appeal to you therefore brethren, by the mercies of God, to present your bodies as a living sacrifice, holy and acceptable to God, which is your spiritual worship."

Romans 12:1 ESV

"Do you not know that you are God's temple and that God's spirit dwells in you? If anyone destroys God's temple, God is destroy him. For God's temple is holy, and you are that temple."

1 Corinthians 3:16-17 CSB

"And do not get drunk with wine, for that is debauchery, but be filled with the spirit."

Ephesians 5:18 ESV

Practice What You Preach

1. List and provide details of 10 ways that you can improve your temple.

    1. _____
    2. _____
    3. _____
    4. _____
    5. _____
    6. _____
    7. _____
    8. _____
    9. _____
    10. _____

2. List some hobbies or activities you can do to help improve your temple.

3. List things you want to learn, and how you will go about learning them this year to better yourself.

12

Don't Stress Over Things You Can't Control

"Peace I leave with you, my peace I give to you: not as the world gives, give I unto you. Let not your heart be troubled, neither let it be afraid."

John14:27 KJB

How many times does the phrase "Fear not" occur in the Bible? The answer will surprise you. It's not a small number. It is not just a handful of times. It actually appears in the Bible 365 times. That's a "Fear not" for every day of the year! What does that tell us about worry and anxiety? It tells us that even God doesn't want us to worry and fear. The scripture asks, can we add one day to our life worrying about the future?

Actually, we can take days away from our life if we worry too much. The term "worry yourself to death" is not just a euphemism. Stress, anxiety, and worry produce increased stress hormones (cortisol, epinephrine, norepinephrine, etc.) in our bodies, which can actually clog our arteries, leading to heart attacks and strokes. It can also slow down blood flow, resulting in the decreased function of our organs, reducing the luster and resiliency of our skin. It can cause damage to organs like the spleen, liver, and kidneys, whose job is to filter the blood; when those organs work harder, they can fail sooner than the natural progression of deterioration in the body. Stress slows down our cognitive function and ability to concentrate. It causes worry lines and an aged appearance. It makes us feel fatigued and run down, causing impairments in our sleep. Stress can contribute to other health problems like diabetes, obesity, and blood pressure. It can cause headaches, tension, and migraines. It can affect our stomachs and digestion, resulting in irritable bowel and inflammation in the gut. It can change our sex drives and androgen (hormone) levels, resulting in erectile dysfunction and female sexual arousal disorder. It can cause chest pain, muscle pain, joint pain, and exacerbate fibromyalgia and chronic pain. It can cause trouble with your appetite, resulting in under or overeating, which can change your nutrition status and weight.

With stress having all of these possible impacts on our body, it is no wonder that God beseeches us to not worry or stress so many times throughout the Bible. The first step in treating any condition, including too much stress, is acknowledging that there is a problem and identifying the causes so that they can be addressed. We must realize that there are two types of stressors: negative stressors that come from events that will typically have a poor or negative outcome, and positive stressors from events that typically have a good or positive outcome. The major negative stressors are typically caring for our basic needs, job and career issues, school grades and performance, trauma (emotional, physical, sexual), world issues and listening to the news, family issues like separation and divorce, and dealing with death. The difficulty in dealing with stress is that it doesn't come separately, in fact it usually comes all at once, piling up and weighing us down. You've heard of the saying, "When it rains it pours?" This is typically because things seem to pile up all at once: you go through a divorce, get depressed, get sick, have to go to the hospital, lose your job, and then bills are due all at once.

People associate stress with negative events, but positive events can be stressful as well. If you've ever planned a party or a wedding, you know the stress of dealing with invitations, seating arrangements, food, entertainment, and paying for it all. On the evening of my wedding, I was so tired and ready for the day to be over! It was one of the best days of my life, but acting as referee to feuding family members, paying vendors, taking pictures, and trying to spend time with each guest was so overwhelming.

Other positive events that can cause stress include having a new relationship or going on a date, having a baby, meeting a deadline, winning a sporting competition, and planning a vacation. , Large changes in your way of living like buying a house, starting or graduating from college, getting a promotion, and even winning the lottery can cause stress. Even though these events are positive and welcomed by most, they disrupt the normal way of life, and that disruption can be overwhelming.

Stress is regular part of life. We cannot eliminate stress, but we can learn to manage it. The first step in managing stress is to recognize what triggers it, and deal with it early when it occurs. We handle stress better by talking with someone like a therapist, counselor, doctor, or life coach. There are also options like engaging in relaxation techniques, keeping a diary or journaling, and learning how to better manage your time. One of my favorite ways of dealing with stress, I have already discussed extensively, and you can probably guess. Exercise! I love to go for a brisk walk, attend a kickboxing class, go to a dance class like Zumba, or lift weights when I'm feeling stressed. I often envision that the situations causing me stress are on the punching bag, and I take out my frustrations on the bag.

Another way I've learned to manage stress is by not voluntarily taking on new stress when possible, and learning to say NO. Its ok to say no when people are asking you to take on more tasks when you're already feeling tired and burnt out. You will not be any less of a person or hero if you say no. In fact, you'll be a hero to yourself by promoting self-care, awareness, and a healthy lifestyle by not taking on more than you can handle. We must mentally put away the notion of being a superhero. We are human and that is ok!

Sometimes we need to disconnect from the world around us to deal with stress. The constant barrage of negative news, online access to everything, and social media can cause undue stress. I've had patients who required medication because they watched the world news, and felt so forlorn and in despair with what is going on in our world that it started to negatively affect their health. Disconnecting, turning off the television, not reading the news, logging off from our social media accounts, and not checking emails is sometimes very necessary for our mental and physical health.

Conversely, we must also know when there is a need to connect. Sometimes being too disconnected, isolated, and alone can be depressing and cause stress. No man is an island, and there are times when the company of others can help us through situations. Good feelings and positive reactions come from healthy relationships and interactions with others. Joining a social club with members that are similar to you, or playing with a team of likeminded individuals, is a great way to connect. Finding a therapist or life coach is also a good way to connect with others. Spending more time with family is also a great way to deal with stress.

Perhaps the best way to manage stress is to rest. We must give our bodies the rest it requires. So many times, we are burning the candle at both ends thinking that it is necessary for progress. But all it does is burn us in the end. I often tell my patients, if you don't take a break or rest, your body will take a rest for you, and that can have dire consequences like major illness, hospitalizations, and even death. In this same vein, we must ensure we are getting enough sleep so that we can better handle and manage all the stressors we face on a daily basis. Sleep allows the body to reset and renew itself on a cellular level, but it also renews our minds.

Good sleep has cycles: REM (rapid eye movement) sleep, and non-REM sleep. Most sleep cycles occur in about 90 minutes, and good, effective sleep cycles multiple times. This can't be done in 4-5 hours, so although you are busy, it is imperative that you get sleep. Adults are recommended to get 8 hours of sleep each night, teens 8-10 hours, and children require 10-12 hours.

This brings us to a great point. Even children and teens deal with stress and need to be allowed to acknowledge and manage their stress in healthy ways as well. Many adults brush off teen and childhood feelings, assuming that children simply don't understand a particular situation due to their young age. I've heard parents tell their children to just be quiet, that they don't know what they're talking about, and that they're too young to understand. But this is farthest from the truth. Children and teens have feelings that can be hurt, and they have neurotransmitters that can be off balance as much, if not more than, adults. Because children's brains are still developing, they can get surges of chemical imbalance, leading to sudden displays of aggression or emotions. Children deal with school, peer pressure, chores, studying, sports, body changes and body image, sibling rivalry, separation anxiety, and taking on their parent's or caregiver's stress. Teens deal with body image, grades, college prep, tryouts, and deal with parents and siblings. They face some of the same issues their parents faced growing up like peer pressure, and parents can relate to some of the issues. Unfortunately, teens now have the problem of online bullying that their parents probably never dealt with, so navigating the process can be daunting and scary. Teens and children need to be allowed to acknowledge and manage their stress as well.

One thing to keep in mind, for all ages, is to not add more stress on top of already stressful situations. The ways that we address or attempt to manage our stress should be healthy and not excessive. Though a glass of wine may help to relax you, drinking too much has negative consequences. One should avoid drinking too much alcohol or caffeine, engaging in any drug use, or smoking cigarettes to deal with stress, as these are not healthy and cause more problems in the long run.

The last suggestion in dealing with stress is to take control of your situation. Do not allow your circumstances to control you. Sometimes situations seem impossible to solve, but instead of letting this worry you or cause stress, take a break, then come back with a clear head and find other ways of tackling the problem. With large tasks, taking one small piece at a time can make the task more manageable, making it easier to overcome. Try to find multiple solutions to solving problems so that if one way does not work, you have other ideas. How do you eat a whale? One bite at a time! How do you handle stress? One small healthy solution at a time, until the problem or situation causing the stress is handled.

Meditate Day and Night

"Remove vexation from your heart, and put away pain from your body, for youth and the dawn of life are vanity."

Ecclesiastes 11:10 ESV

"Let not your heat be troubled: you believe in god, believe also in me. In my Father's house are many mansions: if it were not so, I would have told you. I go to prepare a place for you. And if I go and prepare a place for you, I will come again, and receive you to myself; that where I am, there you may be also. And where I go you know, and the way you know."

John 14:1-4 NAS

"Are not two sparrows sold for a penny? Yet not one of them will fall to the ground outside your Father's care. And even the very hairs of your head are all numbered So don't be afraid; you are worth more than many sparrows."

Matthew 10:29-30 NIV

"Do not be anxious about anything, but in every situation, by prayer and petition, with thanksgiving, present your requests to God."

Philippians 4:6 NIV

"Cast all your anxiety on him because He cares for you."

1 Peter 5:7 BSB

"For God has not given us the spirit of fear, but of power, and of love, and a sound mind."

2 Timothy 1:7 KJV

"You keep him in perfect peace whose mind is stayed on you, because he trusts in you"

Isaiah 26:3 ESV

"Therefore I tell you, do not worry about your life, what you will eat or drink; or about your body, what you will wear. Is not life more than food, and the body more than clothes? Look at the birds of the air; they do not sow or reap or store away in barns, and yet your Heavenly Father feeds them. Are you not much more valuable than they? Can any one of you by worrying add a single hour to your life? And why do you worry about clothes? See how the flowers of the field grow. They do not labor or spin. Yet I tell you that not even Solomon in all his splendor was dressed like one of these. If that is how God clothes the grass of the field, which is here today and tomorrow is thrown into the fire, will he not much more clothe you- you of little faith So do not worry, saying 'what shall we eat?' or 'what shall we drink?' or 'what shall we wear?" For the pagans run after all these things, and your heavenly Father knows that you need them. But seeks first His kingdom and his righteousness, and all these things will be given to you as well. Therefore do not worry about tomorrow, for tomorrow will worry about itself. Each day has enough trouble of its own."

Matthew 6:25-34 NIV

Practice What You Preach

1. Identify 10 negative situations that cause you stress.

    1. _____
    2. _____
    3. _____
    4. _____
    5. _____
    6. _____
    7. _____
    8. _____
    9. _____
    10. _____

2. Identify 10 positive situations that cause you stress.

    1. _____
    2. _____
    3. _____

4. _____

5. _____

6. _____

7. _____

8. _____

9. _____

10. _____

3. List some healthy ways you can deal with your stressors.

4. Plan to disconnect from social media and negative news for a few hours each week. List some other things you can do during the time you would usually engage in social media, email, news, etc.

5. List specific people in your life who you can connect with to improve and lower stress levels (family, therapist, doctor, life coach, etc.)

Conclusion

Now that you have learned the 12 secrets to divine health, the next step is to practice what you preach. If you have not already done so, go back and fill out the practice what you preach section after each chapter to put into practice the suggestions to help you improve your overall health. Your health and wellness are vital to your future, your children's and family's future, and the well-being of your community! I truly wish a 3 John 2 and John 10:10 life for each of you; prosper in good health, even as your souls prosper, and live life more abundantly!

Thank You

I'd like to thank Pastor Al and all the other Pastors and ministers who selflessly attend to the spiritual, mental, and overall health and wellness of others. Who is Pastor Al you ask? He is a 45-year-old pastor of a nondenominational church, with 150 to 200 members. He is married with three children ranging in age from 8 to 19. He works full-time as an electrician in his own business. He devotes a great deal of time to the ministry, leading and spearheading various ministries, including the Couple's Ministry, Teen Outreach, Choir (as he is a musician himself), Community Outreach, and the Evangelism Team. He is also the Assistant Coach of a little league football team, and tries to be active in his children's lives and extracurricular activities. He loves and adores his wife, and wished he could spend more time with her. Unfortunately, due to his busy schedule, he saw her briefly after coming home and before he went to bed. They tried to go on a date at least once a month to catch up and have some fun, but these dates were few and far between. Then Pastor Al attended a conference for pastors where the speaker discussed the health and wellness of pastors. That's when Pastor Al realized he hadn't been to see a doctor since he was diagnosed with a minor illness a few years ago. He had not even had a physical. Pastor Al began thinking to himself, how am I promoting spiritual wellness in everyone, when I'm not caring for my temple?

He started to wonder how he would find the time to see a doctor between his full work schedule, full-time ministry, Community work, and family. He decided that the doctor would have to wait until he found time, after all, he felt healthy. The occasional burning in his chest was simply heartburn. Right? The 50 pounds he gained over the past five years would come off when he found time to get back in the gym. right?

Pastor Al realized at that conference that he gave so much that he neglected his own health. He thought of the colleagues he knew who had to stop pastoring due to health issues, and some of the ones that had strokes or amputations from uncontrolled diabetes. He decided to make a change in his life so that he could be better equipped to care for others.

Pastor Al is fictional, but I know so many pastors just like him. Pastor Al became the blueprint for my new medical practice, Abundant Life Concierge, which cares for pastors, and helps them manage their health and wellness.

If you'd like to learn more about Abundant Life Concierge, and how Dr. Nicole can help you better care for yourself while you care for others, follow her on all social media:

Website: www.drnicoledo.com

Facebook: www.facebook.com/drnicoledo

Twitter: @drnicoledo

Instagram: @drnicoledo

LinkedIn: www.linkedin.com/drnicoledo

Schedule a discovery session to learn more about her services at pastorscare.com or by calling (803)543-2913

SOURCES

Scriptures marked AMP are taken from the Amplified Version®. Copyright © 2015 by The Lockman Foundation. All rights reserved.

Scriptures marked ASV are taken from the American Standard Version. All rights reserved.

Scriptures marked ESV are taken from English Standard Version®. Copyright © 2001 by Crossway, a publishing ministry of Good News Publishers. All rights reserved.

Scriptures marked MSG are taken from The Message®. Copyright © 1993, 1994, 1995, 1996, 2000, 2001, 2002. Used by permission of NavPress Publishing Group.

Scriptures marked NASB are taken from the New American Standard Bible®. Copyright © 1960, 1962, 1963, 1968, 1971, 1972, 1973, 1975, 1977, 1995 by The Lockman Foundation. Used by permission.

Scriptures marked NIV are taken from the New International Version®. Copyright © 1973, 1978, 1984, 2011 by Biblica, Inc.™. All rights reserved.

Scriptures marked NKJV are taken from the New King James Version®. Copyright © 1982 by Thomas Nelson. All rights reserved.

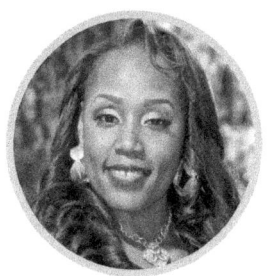

About the Author

Dr. Nicole Edwards is a practicing board-certified family medicine physician in Columbia, SC. She received her doctorate in osteopathic medicine from the New York College of Osteopathic Medicine and also holds two masters' degrees in professional counseling and marriage and family therapy.

Currently, Dr. Edwards works as a traveling physician and medical director for True Counsel Behavioral Health. She also serves as assistant medical director for Heartstrings Hospice. Her mission includes helping busy working professionals, pastors, and congregants to transform their mind, body, and spirit. Her dedication to helping others achieve whole-man-health-and-wellness led to the inception of Abundant Life Concierge, where she specializes in health and wellness for pastors and congregations, and provides personalized medical care to the community.

To learn more, visit her website at www.drnicoledo.com

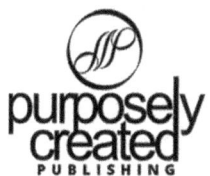

CREATING DISTINCTIVE BOOKS WITH INTENTIONAL RESULTS

We're a collaborative group of creative masterminds with a mission to produce high-quality books to position you for monumental success in the marketplace.

Our professional team of writers, editors, designers, and marketing strategists work closely together to ensure that every detail of your book is a clear representation of the message in your writing.

Want to know more?
Write to us at info@publishyourgift.com
or call (888) 949-6228

Discover great books, exclusive offers, and more at
www.PublishYourGift.com

Connect with us on social media

@publishyourgift

www.ingramcontent.com/pod-product-compliance
Lightning Source LLC
Chambersburg PA
CBHW071629080526
44588CB00010B/1333